P·R·A·T·I·C·A·L
PARENTING

A–Z Guide
to Children's
Health

Dr David H

First published in Great Britain in 1999
by Metro Books (an imprint of Metro Publishing Limited),
19 Gerrard Street, London W1V 7LA

Edited by Penelope Cream
Consultant Editor Anne Hunt
Illustrations by Kate Simunek

British Library Cataloguing in Publication Data. A CIP record of this book is available on request from the British Library.

ISBN 1 900512 68 8

10 9 8 7 6 5 4 3 2 1

Typeset by Wakewing, High Wycombe, Buckinghamshire
Printed in Great Britain by Caledonian, Glasgow

Contents

How to Use This Book

If your child is ill or has an accident, you need clear, accurate information. You need to know what to do, and how urgently you need to do it.

To help you, the topics in this book are listed alphabetically, outlining the symptoms, what you can do to alleviate them, and what treatments are available. Some of the problems – such as meningitis and appendicitis – will be emergencies where you need instant information at your fingertips. There is a detailed illustrated section on first aid and emergency resuscitation giving the essential knowledge you might need for more serious situations. Emergencies or cases needing urgent attention are marked with a special symbol.

You may also find this book particularly helpful after you have consulted your doctor. But it is vital to remember that while this book will often give you all the information that you need, there may still be situations when you will still be in doubt. If you are in doubt, then do contact a doctor – it is always better to be safe than sorry.

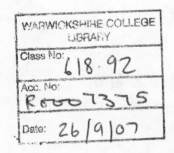

Introduction

It's not easy being a parent. It might be wonderful, thrilling and awe-inspiring, but it can also be a source of real anxiety. There can't be a parent alive who doesn't worry at times about their child's health. Take it from me – even as a doctor I found myself worrying repeatedly about my children when they were young. After all, the world can seem a frighteningly hazardous place. Newspapers are full of tales of meningitis, BSE, scares about immunization, and one new syndrome after another. Caring parents need information more than ever.

Few of us feel sufficiently prepared when our first child arrives. Tiny babies seem so frail, and new parents are bound to feel worried and concerned, and worried about being over-concerned. It can seem so dreadfully difficult to get the balance right. After all, how do you know whether you are being too anxious about each and every sniffle and cough, or whether you are ignoring symptoms that might be the start of a really dangerous illness like meningitis or something even worse? New parents can feel that they are expected to become instant experts in diagnosis and treatment. It can be very daunting.

Having clear information at your fingertips can make all the difference to how confident you feel. Confidence can be something that many young parents lack. In years gone by, most young parents had their own parents living nearby. Today, new parents often have no one other than health-care professionals to turn to when they are worried or concerned – and then they worry about being a nuisance. It feels like they just can't win!

This book is designed to give parents a lot of information in an easily accessible form. It will unravel the serious from the minor, and point you in the right direction when it comes to knowing how to care for your child. I really do hope that you find it useful. Parents need all the help they can get.

David Haslam

The Home Medicine Chest

All parents need a simple supply of medication to use when their child is ill.

You may think that you need a wide variety of medicines, ready for when your child suffers from a sore throat, tummy upset, cough, cold, or some other ailment. In fact, you are much better to have a small simple supply of treatments that you understand, and know when and how to use them. I would simply recommend that you keep the following:

- Paracetamol medicine (such as Calpol or Disprol)

- Paracetamol tablets for older children and adults

- Rehydration sachets for diarrhoea (such as Rehidrat or Dioralyte) – be sure to follow the recommended dosage

- Calamine lotion for itching, rashes or bites

- For babies: cream to prevent nappy rash, such as zinc and castor oil

- An antihistamine, such as Piriton, can be helpful for any form of itch or allergy

- Plasters and sterile dressings

I suspect that this short list may come as a surprise. In fact, these are the only 'over the counter' medicines that my wife and I ever used for our own children throughout their entire childhood. Obviously, if your child has some long-term medical problem such as asthma or eczema, you will also need the relevant drugs that your GP prescribes or advises, but this simple selection is aimed at the average family, and should cover most important everyday medical needs.

While paracetamol is generally the most commonly prescribed and used pain-killer for children, ibuprofen (also called Nurofen, Brufen or Cuprofen) can also be extremely effective, although it is not usually the best choice of prescription for children with asthma.

USING 'OVER THE COUNTER' MEDICINES

I realize that many parents will also want to purchase other treatments such as cough medicines. When you buy any medicine, do make sure that the pharmacist knows the age of your child, as there are usually different formulations for different ages. There are also some simple rules for using medication that you should always try to follow:

● Make sure that you know exactly what the dose is, and how often it should be given – and make sure that you use the spoon provided. Most doses are measured in 5ml spoons. If you use a teaspoon, you may be giving a smaller dose than is recommended or needed. Measuring syringes, available from all pharmacists, are much more accurate to use.

● Do ask if the medicine has any side-effects. Some antihistamines and cough medicines can make children sleepy. You will worry less if you know what to expect.

● Check the expiry date on any medicines in your medicine cabinet. Any that are out of date should be returned to the pharmacist if you can't be certain that you can dispose of them safely.

● Make sure that any medicines that you keep in the house are firmly locked away. Don't simply leave them on a shelf, or in an unlocked cupboard where your child might be able to get hold of them. Medication may often come in childproof bottles, but many children find these easier to open than adults do.

GIVING YOUR CHILD MEDICATION

No parent ever enjoys giving medicine to a child. Sometimes it can be a real battle, even with medicines that have been designed to taste as pleasant as possible. Trying to slip a spoon between clenched gums while your child is shaking his head from side to side can test the patience of any parent – particularly when you yourself end up covered in a spoonful of sticky antibiotic. A 5ml spoonful can cover an awful lot of clean shirt.

However, there are ways in which you can make giving medicines less of a stressful chore. Try the following tips and suggestions:

- Most medicines for children are prescribed as liquid suspensions or syrups. Ask your pharmacist if you can have an oral dosage syringe. This is provided with an adaptor that fits into the top of the medicine bottle, and the syringe is marked in 0.5ml divisions from 1 to 5ml in case you need to give dosages of less than 5ml.

- When giving medicines using a dosage syringe, make sure your child is sitting up. Simply aim into the side of the mouth, and push the plunger down very slowly. Try not to squirt the medicine at high speed into the back of your child's throat, or he or she will almost certainly gag as a result.

- Remember that trying to give medicines to a child who is lying down can be dangerous, as the child may inhale rather than swallow.

- The design for many of the spoons provided free with many medicines is completely hopeless. The dose is only accurate when the spoon is full, but it is almost completely impossible to give a spoonful without spilling the contents.

- There are a number of commercially available spoons with a sensible lip to them, so if you don't use a dosage syringe, consider buying one of these.

- Your own attitude to the medicine can make a tremendous difference. If you give the impression that a medicine is bound to be unpleasant, then your child is bound to react unfavourably.

- Try to avoid bribery, as in 'if you take this, you can have some sweets'. Children are not stupid. If bribery is needed, they will assume the experience is going to be unpleasant.

- You may find it easier to transfer a spoonful of medicine into a small cup, and then give a little bit at a time. This way, if any is spat out it can be collected and given again. However, it isn't wise to put medicine into a large volume of drink as it may not all be taken. Instead, if necessary, have a drink on offer to give as soon as the medicine is finished.

- If your child really does find a particular medicine completely unpalatable, have a word with your doctor to see if there is an alternative preparation available that has a more pleasant taste.

EAR DROPS

When giving ear drops, lie your child on his or her side, or else tilt the head away from the side in which you want to put the drops. Hold the dropper close to the ear and gently squeeze the rubber bulb, releasing the drops into the ear canal, then leave the child in this position for a couple of minutes. Repeat this on the other side if necessary.

NOSE DROPS

In babies, it is best to lie your baby face up across your knee with her neck resting on your thigh. Gently support the head with one hand, put the dropper inside the nostril and release the necessary number of drops, then repeat in the other nostril. You might persuade an older child to blow his or her nose first. Then she should lie down face up, with her neck resting on a bunched up pillow and her head tilted backwards. It is easy to insert the drops in this position. Wait a minute or so before letting your child get up again so that the drops do not run out.

EYE DROPS

It is usually best to have help when trying to put drops into your child's eye, unless he or she is remarkably co-operative. One of you should hold the head steady while the other holds the dropper in one hand, resting this hand against the child's forehead. Now, with the index finger of the other hand, gently pull the lower eyelids downwards. Then gently release the drops into the area between the eye and the lower eyelid. Do not touch the eye with the dropper.

If you are using an eye ointment, use a similar technique, again rolling the lower lid downwards and squeezing a small amount of the ointment along the inside of the eyelid – just like squeezing toothpaste onto a toothbrush. Your child will then blink, and the blinking will spread the ointment over the whole surface of the eye.

Safety in the Home

It is well known that more accidents happen in the home than anywhere else. What can seem a safe and happy environment can contain all manner of hazards, and these become more obvious when your child starts to become mobile. Follow these guidelines:

THE KITCHEN
- Keep bleach and other chemicals well out of reach, ideally in a locked cupboard. Ensure all chemicals are labelled clearly.
- Never leave saucepan handles overhanging the edge of the cooker.
- Keep knives well out of reach.
- Make sure the flex of the iron is well out of your child's way.

THE BATHROOM
- Never ever leave your child unattended in the bath.
- Run the water before you put your child in, and do check the temperature.
- Keep all medicines, chemicals and razors well out of reach.

THE GARDEN
- If you have pets, make sure that any faeces are cleaned up straight away. Keep sandpits well covered.
- Cover garden pools, or make sure that your child cannot possibly fall into them.
- Teach your child that it is not safe to eat anything at all straight from the garden.

THE BEDROOM
- Never use a pillow for a baby under one year of age.
- Make sure that cupboards can be opened from the inside.
- Never put your child to bed with anything round his or her neck.
- In all rooms, ensure that electrical equipment is unplugged when not in use, and use plug safety covers.

Getting the Best Out of Your Doctor

In the UK it is likely that parents of young children will consult their doctor many times each year. Your relationship with your doctor should be a real partnership, and there is a lot that you both can do to help the relationship work. Having a doctor that you trust can make an enormous difference to a family.

There are two main occasions when you will need to contact a GP. There will be the routine appointments, the check-ups, and the minor anxieties. For these, do get to know how your practice works. It may be more appropriate for you to see a nurse practitioner, practice nurse, or health visitor for many childhood problems. Ask the receptionists for advice about who to see.

And then there are the emergencies when you need advice and help NOW. Throughout the book I will be giving very clear guidelines about when you do need urgent medical help, but don't hesitate to seek medical advice if ever you are concerned about your child.

Many doctors and practices are now very happy to give advice on the telephone. If the problem is an absolute desperate emergency, then ask for help straight away. In most cases, though, if the doctor or nurse is busy when you call and you simply want advice, he or she will phone you back.

CALLING THE DOCTOR

When you telephone your surgery or health centre you need to be ready with some clear information. The doctor and practice team receive a large number of different calls throughout the day, and they need to be able to put them into some order of priority. So be ready with

- Your name and address

- Your phone number

- Your child's name

- What appears to be wrong with your child

- How urgent you believe the problem is

- Whether you need a home visit or just telephone advice

- Whether you need to speak to the doctor now, or whether it can wait

When you consult the doctor, don't be disappointed if you don't come away with a prescription. Most childhood illnesses are viral infections and these are not helped in any way by antibiotics, or indeed by anything other than paracetamol. If your doctor recommends simple measures such as paracetamol or fluids for your child's illness, it really does not mean that your problem has not been taken seriously, or that the doctor does not understand how worried you are. It simply means that medication will do nothing to help speed your child's recovery.

Outside routine surgery hours, more and more doctors now work in out-of-hours 'doctors' co-ops'. These are groups of trained GPs who share on-call duties, and are often based at an out-of-hours medical centre. Doctors are no longer obliged by their contract to visit other than for medical reasons, and you may well be asked to transport your child to see the doctor. There are many advantages to this system. The doctor you will see will be fresh, and working in a fully staffed and equipped medical centre. While patients and parents often yearn for access to their 'own' doctor available on call for them 24 hours a day, every day, the volume of out-of-hours work means that this is frequently no longer possible, nor safe. However, one side-effect of the increasing use of 'co-ops' is that the doctor you see will not have access to your child's medical records. So, when you speak to the doctor on the phone or attend the out-of-hours centre, do make sure the doctor you see knows about any allergies or significant past medical problems.

And most important of all – if a doctor tells you something you don't understand, then ask questions. It's your child. You need to know.

A-Z
Guide

Allergies

See also Asthma ● Conjunctivitis, Allergic ● Diet ● Hayfever ● Urticaria

Allergies are becoming increasingly common. Whenever a potentially harmful chemical comes into contact with the body, the body immediately produces protective chemicals. In an allergy, the body mistakes a usually harmless substance for a harmful one and the protective reaction occurs unnecessarily. Any substance that triggers off this reaction is called an allergen, and the range of possible allergens is vast – ranging from pollens and pets to house dust mites, drugs or foods.

Allergies run in families. If both parents have allergies, there is a two-in-three chance that their children will have allergies too. If one parent has allergies and the other does not, then the children have a 25–50 per cent chance of being allergic. If neither parent has allergies, the risk of the child being allergic is around 10 per cent.

SYMPTOMS

These depend on the part of the body involved, but the mechanism is the same everywhere. The child initially develops antibodies to a particular substance. These antibodies are found in the lining of the nose, throat, lungs, gut and the skin. When the allergen and the antibodies come into contact with each other, another chemical called histamine is released and it is this that causes the symptoms of an allergic reaction to be produced. If the allergy is in the nose, then the lining of the nose swells up, and the nose runs. If the problem is in the lungs, an attack of asthma may be triggered. In the skin, urticaria (or hives) may result, while bowel allergies may produce nausea, vomiting, abdominal pain and diarrhoea.

Allergies

SYMPTOMS *continued*

FOOD ALLERGIES

A number of symptoms may be linked with a food allergy, though it is important to remember that all these symptoms have many other possible causes. These reactions sometimes occur within minutes of eating a so-called 'trigger' food. Common symptoms include eczema, hayfever, asthma, headache (including migraine), abdominal pains, diarrhoea, acute swellings or tingling of the mouth, lip or tongue, urticaria, vomiting, bloated stomach, runny nose, and even acute anaphylactic shock, which is life-threatening and requires immediate medical attention (see below). The foods that are most often the cause of allergies are milk, egg, wheat, cheese, fish, shellfish, chocolate, tomato, soya, citrus fruits and yeast. If a particular symptom is caused by a food allergy, it will occur on every occasion your child eats that food. If it only occurs sometimes, then it is not an allergy.

ACTION

A severe reaction to an allergen can be very serious and in rare cases results in **anaphylactic shock**. Anaphylactic reactions occur chiefly with allergies where the allergen can get to all parts of the body very rapidly. This mainly occurs with insect bites or stings, or with certain food allergies – particularly eggs, fish, cow's milk protein and nuts (particularly peanuts).

The symptoms of anaphylactic shock include:

- Raised rash on entire body
- Swelling of the face and eyelids
- Swollen lips
- Swollen tongue
- Possible wheezing
- Feeling faint
- Diarrhoea

The child needs an immediate injection of adrenaline. Call both 999 and a doctor immediately. If this has already happened to your child once, your doctor may have given you a supply of adrenaline to inject your child

Allergies

ACTION *continued*

yourself. While waiting, try to give your child a dose of antihistamine using an oral dosage syringe if you have one. Stay with your child, trying your very hardest to keep him or her calm. Fear and panic greatly worsen the situation. If by any chance your child stops breathing, do not hesitate to perform CPR (cardio-pulmonary resuscitation) immediately (see the **First Aid** section pages 93–105).

Less severe forms of allergy are not an emergency, but you should still consult your doctor for advice and treatment, as antihistamines may be useful. As a general rule, your child should avoid coming into contact with the cause of the allergy wherever possible. If the cause of the reaction is in doubt, your child can be given a skin, or patch, test, when small amounts of allergens are placed on the skin to try to identify which substances he or she may be sensitive to.

FOOD ALLERGIES

Sometimes it will be obvious that your child has a food allergy. If your child comes out in a dramatic rash every time he eats eggs, for example, then the diagnosis is clear-cut. It can be much less easy to sort out the possibility of allergy related to other conditions. Some children, for instance, keep getting ear infections. Sometimes, though infrequently, this can be the result of an allergy to cow's milk, but usually it is not. To unravel this you should start by consulting your family doctor who may seek the advice of a paediatrician or dietician. If your suspicions of allergy are strong, keep a diary of symptoms and food intake. It may be possible to spot a link between foods that were taken before a specific symptom occurred. Skin tests are rarely particularly helpful since a positive reaction to a skin test does not necessarily prove the existence of a food allergy.

Perhaps the simplest way to confirm an allergy is to withdraw that particular food from your child's diet. For simple allergies to single foods this can be straightforward, but for more complex possibilities such as dairy product allergies you need detailed advice from an expert, and your doctor should be able to put you in touch with a qualified and interested dietician. If your child suffers from conditions such as eczema or migraine, it is well worth getting

ACTION *continued*

more information on possible dietary triggers from your doctor or health visitor. Don't cut out important foods like dairy products without consulting your GP or health visitor.

USUAL TREATMENT

The level of treatment needed depends on the severity of the allergy. For more serious reactions which can cause anaphylactic shock, such as peanut allergy, your child needs emergency drugs. Treatment in less serious cases involves providing liquid antihistamines, which block the effect of histamine, and also avoiding the substances that your child is allergic to. This is not always easy. Children who are allergic to nuts have to be particularly careful as nut products can turn up in all sorts of unexpected foodstuffs. The parents of children with severe food allergies need to become expert in reading food labels.

If you already have a child with food allergies, and want to try to minimize the risk in subsequent children, there is evidence that the longer you can avoid introducing foods that your baby might be allergic to, the better this is. There is evidence that while the intestines are immature they are not so good at filtering out or digesting potentially allergenic foodstuffs. Some foods are more likely to trigger allergies than others, so when you start to introduce solids you should begin with the least risky foods. These are bananas, carrots, rice and barley cereals and mashed potatoes. Avoid packaged foods if you can as, if an allergy does develop, then it will be much harder to know what foodstuffs are to blame. In addition, try to avoid citrus fruits such as oranges and lemons, egg yolk before nine months, and egg white before one year.

Anaemia

See also Coeliac Disease ● Diet

Anaemia means that the blood is weaker than normal, usually due to a shortage of iron resulting in low levels of haemoglobin, a chemical that carries oxygen around the body.

SYMPTOMS

A child with anaemia will probably be pale and unusually tired and may sometimes have headaches. If the anaemia is severe, even moderate exercise can cause breathlessness.

ACTION

There are different types of anaemia, but to make sure that your child's diet is not the cause, include a variety of the following sources of iron: meat, wheat, beans, lentils, wholemeal flour, dried fruit, leafy green vegetables and egg yolk. If you suspect your child is anaemic, consult your doctor, who will arrange for a blood test to measure the level of haemoglobin in the blood.

USUAL TREATMENT

The treatment depends on the cause.

- A lack of iron in the diet or poor absorption (as in coeliac disease). Your doctor may prescribe iron supplements or liquids.

- An inherited disorder, such as haemolytic or sickle cell anaemia, which may be treated by transfusions or drugs.

- Rarely, bleeding from inside the body, such as in the bowel, is the cause. Treatment depends on finding the bleeding and stopping it.

Anal Fissure

See also Constipation

A potentially painful crack in the skin next to the anus.

SYMPTOMS

An anal fissure is almost always caused by constipation. Passing a hard motion causes the anal skin to crack, and this can cause both pain and slight bleeding. The blood will be bright red and appears either on the nappy or underpants, or else is streaked on the surface of a motion. However, the most significant result of a fissure is worsening constipation. As passing a motion is painful, the child is reluctant to do this, and worsening constipation results. This can become a very vicious circle.

ACTION

While this is certainly not an emergency, if your child does pass any blood do get your doctor to check the problem out.

Make sure that your child's diet includes fresh fruits and vegetables and plenty of fluids to soften faeces.

USUAL TREATMENT

Treatment is aimed at dealing with the constipation. As well as dietary advice, such as the daily inclusion of fruits and fruit juices, your doctor may prescribe a mild laxative. It is important that motions are soft to allow them to be passed comfortably. Your doctor might also prescribe an anaesthetic cream to numb any pain from the fissure.

Antibiotics

Antibiotics are one of the miracles of the past century. Infections that used to kill thousands are now easily overcome. These drugs are easy to take, and those for children are even pleasantly flavoured. But they cannot cure everything.

Many parents still view a consultation with their doctor as a battle to get antibiotics prescribed for their child. They feel let down, or even angry, if the doctor doesn't prescribe them. But the reason that doctors are reluctant to prescribe antibiotics has nothing to do with saving the NHS money, or doctors not understanding how worried parents are. It is much simpler than that. For most childhood infections, antibiotics are useless.

There are two main types of infection: viral infections and bacterial infections. Most sore throats, colds, and even ear infections are caused by viruses. Antibiotics do nothing to help these at all. Even worse, if we use antibiotics indiscriminately, then diseases caused by bacteria will become resistant and much harder to treat. So, doctors may choose not to prescribe them because they *do* care, not because they don't!

However, even though many childhood illnesses need little in the way of treatment other than a cuddle, and perhaps some paracetamol, there are still going to be occasions when your child will need antibiotics. Parents really do need to understand the commonest types, what side-effects they may have, how they should be stored, whether the full course has to be completed, and so on. This section cannot cover every possible antibiotic. After all, in one of the standard reference guides to prescribing for family doctors, known as *MIMS*, there are currently listed 99 different antibiotics. While some of these are the same drug under different names and manufactured by different companies, there are a remarkably large number of entirely different drugs available.

Antibiotics

There are two main groups of antibiotics used in childhood: penicillin and non-penicillin antibiotics. If your child is allergic to the penicillins, then the alternative group will be chosen, and these also have their own particular uses.

EXAMPLES OF COMMONLY PRESCRIBED ANTIBIOTICS:

The same drug may be available under several different names. For example, amoxycillin may be sold under its own name or under a brand name, such as Amoxil, given to it by a drug company.

PENICILLINS

These include Amoxil, amoxycillin, Augmentin, flucloxacillin, Magnapen and Penbritin.

NON-PENICILLIN ANTIBIOTICS

Cephalosporins – such as cefaclor, cephalexin, Ceporex and Distaclor

Macrolides – such as clarithromycin, erythromycin, Erythroped, Klaracid and Zithromax

Others include co-trimoxazole and trimethoprim

Your doctor will choose which antibiotic to use by considering which bacteria are likely to be involved, which antibiotics are most likely to destroy them, how many doses each day need to be given (for example, a dosage of four times a day is tricky with school-age children), and what allergies your child might have. For instance, most urine infections are caused by a bacteria called *E.coli*, which normally inhabits the bowel. Much *E.coli* is now resistant to penicillins, but over 90 per cent of cases can be cured with twice-daily treatment with trimethoprim.

Antibiotics

FORMULATIONS

For children antibiotics are usually given as liquid medicines, though some are available as drops (useful for small babies), or pleasant-flavoured 'chew-tabs' or tablets.

SHOULD THE COURSE BE FINISHED?

Usually your child will need to take a full five- or seven-day course. Do not stop giving the antibiotics when your child feels better as there is a real risk of the bacteria developing resistance to that particular antibiotic so that it will be less effective if needed again. Some bottles contain more medicine than will be needed, so check with your doctor as the prescription is written.

SIDE-EFFECTS

Most antibiotics can cause rashes or diarrhoea. However, most rashes in children on antibiotics are probably not true allergies but are caused by the original infection. Show your doctor or practice nurse the rash rather than assuming an allergy that doesn't exist.

HINTS AND TIPS

- Most antibiotic medicines should be shaken well and stored in the fridge. Check the label.

- Never give antibiotics to other children, however similar the symptoms might be.

- If your child hates the drug's taste, ask for a different flavour.

- If you still have questions, ask your doctor or pharmacist. He or she should always be able to provide full information about any drug that your child might need.

Appendicitis

See also Tummy Ache

Inflammation of the appendix (a blind-ended tube about 7.5cm/3in long, situated at the start of the large intestine) which causes pain in the abdomen.

SYMPTOMS

Parents often worry that abdominal pain is caused by appendicitis, but most tummy aches turn out to be entirely harmless. Typically, appendicitis starts with discomfort around the umbilicus (tummy button). The child then feels sick and the pain shifts to the lower right-hand side of the abdomen and gradually increases in intensity. Most children with appendicitis have a slight fever and typically are reluctant to eat or drink.

ACTION

You should always consult a doctor. Appendicitis can be difficult to diagnose and there isn't a doctor in the world who hasn't been fooled by it, so if pain seems to be getting worse, even if the doctor has said this is not the diagnosis, ask for the pain to be reassessed. If you can't get hold of your doctor, you may need to call an ambulance.

USUAL TREATMENT

The only treatment for appendicitis is admission to hospital for the appendix to be removed in an operation called an appendicectomy. If appendicitis is only suspected, your child may simply be kept in under close observation.

Arthritis

Stiffness, pain, or inflammation affecting one or more joints. Arthritis is more common in adults but can also affect children of any age.

SYMPTOMS

There are several types of arthritis and the main symptoms of each include aching joints, stiffness of the wrist, shoulder or neck, pain in the back, knee, or hip, morning stiffness, loss of appetite and sometimes general tiredness. Arthritis may sometimes follow some other type of infection, such as a sore throat.

ACTION

If a joint is red or swollen, or very painful, then seek help straight away. If generalized joint pains associated with a fever last for more than 24 hours, or if you are concerned that you child may have arthritis, then consult your doctor. You should never try to treat arthritis without having the diagnosis confirmed first.

USUAL TREATMENT

Your GP will almost certainly refer your child to a paediatrician for a detailed assessment. This may include blood tests and x-rays. Treatment will depend on the type and severity of the arthritis and the joints affected, but usually starts with anti-inflammatory medication such as ibuprofen. If just one joint is affected, injection with a steroid can be very helpful in relieving inflammation and pain.

Asthma

This is the most common respiratory disorder of childhood, affecting one in five children. It is caused by inflammation of the lining of the bronchi, the tubes that carry air in the lungs.

SYMPTOMS

The main symptoms of asthma are coughing and/or wheezing. These result from the inflammation of the lining of the bronchi. They are lined with tissue known as mucous membrane which is very similar to the lining of the nose. To understand inflammation, think about what happens when you get a cold and the lining of the nose becomes swollen and congested. Much the same thing can happen with the lining of the air passages in asthma, and the main irritants that can cause symptoms are:

- Infection
- Allergy
- Change of air temperature
- Emotion
- Exercise

For most children, one irritant will be much more important than others, but, whatever the cause, the lining of the bronchi becomes swollen and inflamed and this obstructs the flow of air, causing wheezing or coughing – especially at night. Indeed, your doctor may diagnose asthma even though your child has never seemed to be wheezy.

ACTION

All children who wheeze or have a persistent cough should be assessed by your doctor. If the wheeze is severe – with your child being significantly out of breath – then you should see a doctor right away, but if it is simply a nuisance, then make a routine appointment with your doctor. It may be that your child just wheezes after exercise, or has a wheeze or cough that is worse in the early morning. Both of these can be helped, so don't shy away from consulting a doctor even if the word 'asthma' frightens you. A tremendous amount can be done to control asthma, and a

Asthma

ACTION *continued*

correct diagnosis means that the right treatment can be given, rather than repeated courses of antibiotics or other medication.

If your child is having a bad asthma attack, do not hesitate to call an ambulance.

USUAL TREATMENT

There are two main groups of treatment, preventers and relievers:

RELIEVERS

These include drugs such as Aerolin, Bricanyl, Pulmadil, Salamol, salbutamol, terbutaline and Ventolin. These drugs relieve spasm in the airways in the lungs, and generally work remarkably quickly. They should be used if your child is wheezy, or occasionally may be recommended before exercise. Small babies may not respond to the standard asthma treatments and a drug called Atrovent (ipratropium bromide) may be offered instead until the baby is older.

Reliever drugs may be given as liquid medicines or as various types of inhaler device. Unless your doctor or nurse advises you specifically, these drugs are mainly designed to ease symptoms. Unlike preventer drugs, relievers are used only when necessary.

PREVENTERS

Preventers include drugs such as Aerobec, beclomethasone, Beclazone, Becotide, Flixotide, Intal and Pulmicort. These drugs are known as anti-inflammatories and work by damping down the inflammation of the lining of the airways. For the great majority of asthmatic children these drugs are absolutely essential. Indeed, there is some evidence that the use of relievers alone can actually worsen the inflammation in the bronchi. For all asthmatics, with the exception of children who only wheeze rarely, preventer drugs are vitally important.

These drugs all come as inhalers. Some are given through large transparent plastic devices called large volume spacers (such as

Asthma

Volumatic or Nebuhaler). Others can be given by dry powder inhalers. Your doctor or nurse should be able to go through the options with you to find a treatment that your child is happy to use.

It is absolutely essential that these treatments are used regularly – usually twice every day, until you are advised otherwise. They are almost useless if you simply use them when you think they are needed. Regular use can make a fantastic difference to the severity of the asthma and how well your child feels and sleeps.

SIDE-EFFECTS

Almost all of these drugs consist of tiny doses of steroids (with the exception of Intal), and in general these have very few side-effects provided they are used in the correct doses. They can occasionally cause a thrush infection in the mouth. Intal is virtually free of side-effects and is often used as a first-line preventive treatment, but it is not always effective.

HINTS AND TIPS

- If your child is struggling with any one particular inhaler device, talk to your doctor or nurse. There may be an alternative device which will suit better.

- The chief sign that childhood asthma is not being well enough controlled is usually coughing, not wheezing.

- Remember that there is no such thing as a cure for asthma. The aim of treatment is to keep it under control so that the child lives an entirely normal and active life. The majority of young children with asthma will grow out of it.

- Asthma is not a reason for a child to be any less active than his or her peers.

- It is vital to make your house a no-smoking zone – cigarette smoke is a major irritant.

- Seek urgent help if your child gets breathless despite using his or her usual medication.

Autism and Asperger's Syndrome

Autism is a condition that affects the way a person communicates and relates to other people. Asperger's syndrome is a less severe variant of autism, mainly causing social isolation and eccentric behaviour in childhood.

SYMPTOMS

Symptoms may start to become apparent from the age of three years. Early signs include not fixing his or her eyes on your face, resisting being cuddled, a delay in speaking and, in some cases, hyperactivity. The main problems are difficulties with speech, with non-verbal communication (judging how others are feeling by interpreting the way they look and move), and with social interaction (playing with other children). Children with autism also tend to lack imaginary play (such as pretending a doll is a baby) which normally is an important part of a child's development. However, they tend to have routines and repeated rituals.

ACTION

Autism occurs in just 4 per 10,000 children (more in boys than girls) and Asperger's affects about 26 per 10,000. If you suspect that your child might be autistic, then consult your doctor who will refer your child to a child psychiatrist or psychologist for assessment. Some children have much less severe degrees of autism (described as autistic spectrum disorders).

USUAL TREATMENT

A cure for autism is not known currently but a wide range of therapies and treatments have been developed, which, combined with the right support, treatment and education, help improve the standard of life for a person with autism.

Bedwetting

See also Toilet Training ● Urinary Tract Infection

Night-time toilet training is usually achieved about six months after your child is dry during the day and using a potty easily. Bedwetting should only be considered a problem when a child starts to wet again after being dry, or if the child is not dry by the time he is five.

WHAT TO WATCH FOR

There is no particular age by which all children should be dry at night. Very young children have virtually no bladder control and it is rare for children to have any significant bladder control before they can walk. Approximately 9 out of 10 children become dry at night by the time they are four years old, usually sometime during the third year. The three-year-old may be able to get through the night dry if he is potted at his parents' bedtime.

Control of bowel function comes before control of the bladder, and even after becoming dry all children can temporarily become wet if they are stressed. However, there is certainly no evidence that children who wet their bed have any psychological problems. Physical causes are also unusual, particularly in the child who only wets at night. Children who have problems both during the day as well as at night need closer assessment. The most likely explanation is delayed maturation, which means simply that some children become dry at night later than others, in exactly the same way that some children walk later than others.

ACTION

If you really can't get your child dry at night by the time he is five and you've been down all the potty-training avenues, you will need to seek medical advice. No amount of encouragement will

Bedwetting

ACTION *continued*

make the child mature more quickly. After all, if a child seems late learning to walk, however much you might encourage him, he will only walk when the time is right. However, if your child is occasionally dry at night, then he or she may nearly be ready to become totally dry.

You might want to try a 'star chart'. This is a simple diary chart: every time the child is dry at night he or she puts a coloured star on the appropriate night; for instance, giving the child a blue star for every dry night and a red one for three dry nights in a row. This can be extraordinarily effective – but only when the child is ready and is about to control his bladder. Do not put any undue pressure on your child.

USUAL TREATMENT

If your child is over five years old and still wetting at night, then you should consult a doctor. In addition, you should ask for advice if a child who has previously been dry suddenly becomes wet, or if the child complains of any pain on passing urine, or if it is causing very real upset for either of you.

Initially, the doctor will almost certainly test a urine sample to make sure that there is no infection. Following this, there are a large number of possible treatments or systems to try, such as star charts (as mentioned above), medication and buzzer alarms. None of the treatments is guaranteed as being effective, but most are worth trying.

Many children are not terribly worried about bedwetting, but are concerned if they are going to stay with friends or are going on a trip from school. On these occasions your doctor may prescribe medication, such as Desmospray nasal spray or DDAVP (desmopressin acetate) tablets that interfere with the production of urine overnight. These have no long-term effect, but may give the child confidence and avoid embarrassment.

Bereavement

Children of any age may well have to cope with the death of someone close to them, whether family or friend.

WHAT TO WATCH FOR

After the age of eight years, almost all children have learnt that death is permanent and irreversible. Before this age, their understanding varies enormously. For pre-school and very young children abstract concepts, and particularly religious explanations, may be very confusing. Some children seem to show an extraordinarily sensitive understanding of death; others show no understanding at all, and even assume that whatever happened must have been their fault in some way. This is an entirely logical assumption when you believe that you are the centre of the universe, which is how very small children see their world.

ACTION

If there has been a death in the family, try to keep your child's routine as unchanged as possible. Some children express grief just like adults and they should be encouraged to talk about their feelings. However, others seem to bottle everything up, and if they subsequently seem to be developing physical symptoms or behavioural problems, seek help through your GP.

USUAL TREATMENT

Most children do not need counselling. They simply need love and acceptance, and an opportunity to talk about their feelings. Try to keep talking about the person who has died. If this becomes a taboo subject, albeit inadvertently, this may distress the child very significantly. For children who do seem deeply affected by a death, a child psychologist or counsellor will help by talking to them over a period of time.

Birth Injuries

However much care is taken by the midwife or doctor delivering your baby, a number of birth injuries still occasionally occur.

POTENTIAL PROBLEMS

There are a large number of potential problems. Some will be short term, such as bruising, while others will be much more significant and long term. Bruising is very common just after birth and typically improves over the next few days. Nerve damage can be caused by pressure or bruising on a nerve, and again will usually recover in time. Perhaps the most common example is damage to the nerve that controls the cheek muscles caused by forceps during a forceps delivery. A more serious injury is Erb's palsy, which is caused by stretching or bruising of the nerves in the root of the neck. In this condition the baby may be unable to move the arm and shoulder fully, depending on the nerves involved. Bone fractures rarely occur but if they do the most common injury is a fractured collar bone, which will usually heal without needing treatment.

ACTION

If you are concerned that your child might have suffered any form of birth injury, then consult your doctor who will refer your child for an assessment by a specialist if this seems appropriate.

USUAL TREATMENT

Treatments obviously vary with the injury concerned. In the case of Erb's palsy, for instance, a test called an EMG, or electromyogram, will usually be carried out when your baby is a few weeks old. This test measures electrical activity in the muscle and is used to determine what treatment is needed, which may involve a referral to a paediatric physiotherapist.

Birthmarks

Birthmarks are remarkably common, and are caused by collections of pigment in the skin. The most common varieties are strawberry marks, café au lait spots, freckles and moles.

SYMPTOMS

STRAWBERRY MARKS

These are soft, bright red marks with a raised surface which may appear after birth. They are present at birth in only 1 in 25 babies, but by the age of one year, approximately 1 in 10 children will have one or more. They vary in size from very small to very large, and will usually enlarge significantly over the first six months of life. They will continue to grow more slowly until the age of one year, and then will slowly disappear. Half of all strawberry marks will have disappeared by the age of five, and 90 per cent go by the age of nine years.

CAFÉ AU LAIT SPOTS

These are flat, light brown spots that are the colour of creamy coffee – hence the name – and which are usually bigger than 5mm. They begin to appear shortly after birth. Individually they are harmless, but if there are more than half a dozen this may be the sign of a rare condition known as Von Recklinghausen's disease, an inherited disorder which can cause symptoms affecting hearing and other nervous system problems.

FRECKLES

Freckles are usually less than 5mm in diameter, and are most likely to appear on sun-exposed areas. They usually increase in number as the child gets older and are rarely seen in very young children.

MOLES

These are rare at birth, but the great majority of people will develop moles during their life, with most white people having between 20 and 40 moles by adulthood. Black people will usually have far fewer. Moles are tan, brown or blue-black, and have a regular edge. They tend to get darker as the child gets older.

PORT-WINE STAINS

These are usually purple, flat areas that are caused by a malformation of blood vessels. They often cover a large area but occur singly, most commonly on the face or one of the limbs.

Birthmarks

ACTION

STRAWBERRY MARKS
Most strawberry marks disappear completely, but 1 in 5 might leave some very minor discoloration or slight scarring. However, you should consult your doctor if your child has lots of strawberry marks, or if there is one on the lower part of the back over the spine. In this situation, the mark might possibly be a sign of a spinal problem.

CAFÉ AU LAIT SPOTS
If your child has more than six of these, consult your doctor to rule out Von Recklinghausen's disease.

FRECKLES
Freckles do not matter at all, but if they appear in areas that are not exposed to the sun, then seek your doctor's advice.

MOLES
As your child gets older he or she may have an increasing number of moles. Consult your doctor if any of the moles changes its colour or shape, bleeds or has a different surface appearance from the others.

PORT-WINE STAINS
These seldom fade and, depending on their location, might need to be treated.

USUAL TREATMENT

While strawberry marks and port-wine stains may be unsightly, they only really matter if they are problematic for your child in some way – for instance, a large strawberry mark on an eyelid might make it difficult to see out of that eye. In that sort of situation, laser treatment may help, but this is generally not needed. Most other birthmarks do not need any form of treatment unless they are very unsightly. However, if your child has a mole that is present at birth, or within 14 days of birth, then these have a greater risk of becoming malignant. The risk is small, but these moles should still be assessed by a dermatologist.

Bow Legs

See also Knock-Knees

The shape of the legs caused when the bones curve outwards, producing a larger than normal gap between the knees.

SYMPTOMS

This appearance is the result of the moulding of the bones that takes place while the child is still in the womb. In the vast majority of children their legs gradually straighten out naturally as they get older. Indeed, after the phase of being bowlegged, many children then become knock-kneed before the legs finally straighten up. In a few children, particularly children who are overweight, the bowing may last almost up to the age of four years.

ACTION

If your child seems to be becoming more bowlegged in his or her fourth year, then seek medical advice. Although very few children need surgical correction of the bowing, expert advice is a good idea if the condition persists.

USUAL TREATMENT

Only in exceptional cases will there be a need for any intervention to encourage bowing to straighten out, and even this wouldn't be done in very young children. The initial stage of any medical investigation will simply be monitoring by an orthopaedic consultant. However, if the bowing seems to affect only one leg, seek medical advice right away.

Breath-Holding

See also Convulsions ● Terrible Twos

Breath-holding attacks typically follow a temper tantrum or some other upset, such as a fall.

WHAT TO WATCH FOR

Breath-holding typically starts in the second or third year, and rarely happens after the age of five. If your child is prone to breath-holding, he or she will cry right up to the moment the breath-holding begins, and will then breathe in, and then fail to take another breath. Occasionally the face may go blue, and the arms and legs may seem to jerk.

ACTION

These attacks are frightening, but not dangerous. Your child may possibly become unconscious, but the moment this happens breathing will start again; if it doesn't, perform emergency resuscitation (see page 93), and get urgent help. The vast majority of breath-holding attacks should be treated as temper tantrums and ignored. The more fuss you make, the more they will be repeated, and children need to know that such an attack will not mean that they get their own way.

USUAL TREATMENT

See your doctor if the breath-holding attacks keep happening. Your doctor will examine your child to confirm that nothing else is causing the problem. These attacks normally stop when your child realizes that he or she is being ignored.

Bruising

See also Clotting Disorders

Bruising is marking of the skin, usually blue or purple in colour, and is often the result of a knock. It is caused by blood collecting under the skin from tiny broken blood vessels.

SYMPTOMS

Most bruises follow an injury, which you or your child will be able to identify clearly. Fair-skinned children show bruising more easily, and most bruises take up to two weeks to disappear.

However, if – as rarely happens – bruises appear spontaneously or seem more serious than the injury would seem to warrant, then this can be a sign that the blood is not clotting normally.

ACTION

Minor bruises do not need treatment, but if bruising seems excessive for the type of trauma, then consult your doctor, who will arrange a blood test to rule out rare conditions like leukaemia where bruising sometimes occurs.

USUAL TREATMENT

Simple bruises do not need treatment. With more serious bruising a cold pack may help during the first 12–24 hours. The treatment of spontaneous bruising depends entirely on the cause. The most common problem causing abnormal blood clotting is a condition known as idiopathic thrombocytopenic purpura (ITP) where there are too few platelets in the blood. Frequently it gets better without treatment, but severe cases may need hospital admission or steroid therapy.

Bullying

This usually consists of ongoing targeting of a child by other children, resulting in verbal and sometimes physical abuse.

WHAT TO WATCH FOR

If a child who has previously seemed settled and happy at school becomes reluctant or unhappy to go, then do consider bullying as a possible cause. Children can be very cruel and your child may become picked on, or – perhaps even worse – may become a bully himself. Bullies tend to be children whose parents show little concern for others. They may also lack other outlets for their frustrations and emotions, and may come from extremely strict families.

ACTION

Encourage your child to walk away from the bully, and to take a deliberately low profile. If confrontation seems inevitable, encourage your child to show as little reaction as possible. You could practise this at home. However, don't encourage your child to fight back. This is a recipe for more problems later.

USUAL TREATMENT

Children are frequently frightened and reluctant to say that they are being bullied, so always take complaints about bullies very seriously. Children worry that the bully will find out that he or she has talked, and that the situation will be made worse – so tell your child that you will do nothing without his or her permission. If you can, persuade your child to let you talk to his or her teacher and possibly to the bully's parents.

Cancer

Cancer is one of the diseases that every parent fears, but it is important to remember that it is still extremely rare in children. In the UK only 1 child in 650 will have developed a cancer by the age of 15, and treatment and cure rates are improving all the time. Many childhood cancers can be cured. Cancer occurs in many different forms, depending on the part of the body it affects. It is caused by abnormal growth of cells. The most common types of childhood cancer include leukaemia, which is a cancer of the bone marrow and affects the white blood cells; certain types of brain tumour; neuroblastoma, a cancer of the nervous system; retinoblastoma, a cancer of the retina at the back of the eye; Wilms' tumour, which affects the kidney; and hepatoblastoma, a cancer of the liver.

SYMPTOMS

Since different cancers affect different parts of the body, symptoms vary depending on the organ or tissue area involved. Certain warning signs include tiredness, pale skin, and headaches. Specific symptoms for particular types of cancer may be as follows:

the motions or urine. However, do remember that each of these symptoms can occur on their own and are much more likely to indicate another problem rather than cancer. Talk to your GP about them if you are worried, especially if several symptoms appear together.

LEUKAEMIA
Typical symptoms include anaemia, bruising where your child has not been injured or knocked against anything, nosebleeds, bone or joint pain, swollen glands, swollen red gums, and possibly bleeding in

BRAIN TUMOURS
Possible symptoms may include weakness in the muscles, difficulties with speech, headaches and vomiting. In a small number of cases the child may experience epileptic seizures.

Cancer

NEUROBLASTOMA
This type of tumour affects the nervous system and may appear in the adrenal glands or in the abdomen, occasionally appearing in the neck or chest. Symptoms include general aches and pains, diarrhoea, flushed skin and weight loss.

RETINOBLASTOMA
This cancer appears most commonly in babies and toddlers, rather than in older children. Only one child in 20,000 will suffer from retinoblastoma, which means that it is very rare. It is usually an inherited condition. Symptoms may include poor sight in one eye, leading to a squint and a white-coloured area in the pupil (the black central area).

WILMS' TUMOUR
Also known as a nephroblastoma, this type of cancer affects the kidney and is seen most usually in children under four years. It has an 80 per cent survival rate if treatment is started early. Specific symptoms may include a swelling in the abdomen and sometimes abdominal pain.

HEPATOBLASTOMA
This cancer affects the liver. Typical symptoms include weight loss, tiredness, abdominal pain, loss of interest in food and, in advanced cases, jaundice (yellowing of the skin).

ACTION
The success rates for treatment nowadays are very good, especially when the cancer is treated early. If you are at all worried about your child, then talk to your doctor who will carry out a full examination. If there is a possibility that your child might have cancer, your doctor will arrange an urgent referral to a specialist hospital team for futher investigation.

USUAL TREATMENT

Children with cancer are nearly always treated in hospital by specialist teams. These teams include a number of people, all experts in the treatment of cancer, such as paediatric oncologists (oncology is the study of cancer), pathologists (who examine the cells), haematologists (specialists in blood disorders), radiotherapists and radiologists (who work in the scanning and x-ray departments), and genetic and cancer counsellors.

All these people work together to provide you and your child with as much care, support and information as possible. Do ask them as many questions as you want. The more you know about the condition, the less frightening it may seem. You will also find that the various children's cancer charities (see page 214) are very helpful and can put you in touch with parents whose children have a similar illness. Such support is very helpful.

The hospital team will first carry out various tests to see if the problem is indeed cancer. These include blood tests, ultrasound, CT or MRI scans, x-rays and perhaps a biopsy or lumbar puncture (when a small sample of tissue or spinal fluid is taken for analysis in the laboratory).

The actual treatment of the condition depends on the type of cancer that your child has. The variety of treatments is very wide and is constantly being updated. Once the diagnosis is confirmed, the doctors will decide on the best course of treatment, depending on where the cancer is, what types of cell are involved, and how ill your child is. Generally, cancer treatment usually involves radiotherapy and chemotherapy, when the cells causing the cancer are attacked by x-rays and chemicals. Sometimes surgery will be necessary to examine and perhaps remove the affected area. In the case of leukaemia, blood tranfusions and, sometimes, bone marrow transplants may also be carried out.

Cerebral Palsy

Erratic movement caused by a lack of oxygen or blood flow to the brain either late in pregnancy, or during or after birth.

SYMPTOMS

Approximately one child in 400 has cerebral palsy. The symptoms will depend on which part of the brain was affected. Severe cerebral palsy may be obvious from birth, but lesser degrees may only become apparent later when your child is not able to do the same things as children of the same age. A range of co-ordination difficulties may occur. These include **spasticity**, in which the muscles can be very tight and contract unusually when the child attempts to move; **athetosis**, in which muscles move involuntarily and uncontrollably; **ataxia**, in which balance is poor and walking is very unsteady; and **tremor**, which causes shaking that typically occurs when the child tries to move his or her limbs.

Children are affected to different degrees; not all these symptoms will be seen in every child with cerebral palsy. Some children will have very minor difficulties while others are affected more severely. Nearly half have some difficulty with speech and most will have learning difficulties.

ACTION

If you suspect cerebral palsy, see your GP, who can make a full assessment and refer you to a specialist if necessary.

USUAL TREATMENT

Your child is likely to need specialist physiotherapy and possibly speech therapy. The condition does not worsen with time, but it is vital that children receive continuing attention from their parents, physiotherapists and occupational therapists.

Chest Infections

See also Cold ● Cough ● Croup

Inflammation of the airways in the lungs caused by a bacterial or viral infection.

SYMPTOMS

Most chest infections are preceded by a sore throat, cold or other upper respiratory infection. Typical symptoms include coughing, breathlessness, fever, chest discomfort or offensive breath. A cough will sometimes be phlegmy or loose and sometimes dry. The phlegmy cough is most likely to be caused by some form of infection, while the dry cough may be caused by simple irritation, or may possibly be triggered by asthma. Babies can be particularly distressed by respiratory infections, such as **bronchiolitis**. Bronchiolitis (inflammation of the bronchioles, the smaller airways in the lungs) is a viral infection affecting babies, caused by RSV, or respiratory syncytial virus – the same virus that causes croup in older children. Most common in the first six months, it can affect children up to 18 months old. The symptoms usually start with a cold, a runny nose and possibly a slight fever. However, fairly rapidly the baby becomes wheezy, and this is frequently worse at night.

Infection of the bronchi, the larger air tubes, is very common in children; technically this is known as **bronchitis**. An infection of the actual tissue of the lung as well as the lining of the airways is called **pneumonia**. A child who gets severe or recurrent chest infections may occasionally have an underlying cause such as bronchiectasis, cystic fibrosis or a foreign body (e.g., a peanut) inhaled into one lung. **Bronchiectasis** typically follows an untreated chest infection, or a chest infection associated with a condition such as measles or whooping cough. The walls of the smaller airways are damaged and lose their natural elasticity, resulting in a chronic infection and a very loose cough when an infection is present.

Chest Infections

ACTION

While bronchiolitis is usually a fairly mild condition, it can be severe and if you are concerned that your baby is struggling to breathe, then don't hesitate – seek medical help urgently. Call an ambulance if you can't get your child to hospital yourself. Signs that your baby may be struggling to breathe include rapid breathing, going blue on the lips and around the mouth, drawing in of the space between the ribs and below the lowest ribs, appearing distressed, and tightness of the muscles around the shoulders and neck. In general, if your child seems distressed or breathless, or has a cough associated with a fever, then seek medical help. If your child does not seem particularly unwell, but has a cough that lasts more than three or four days, then it would be a good idea to see your doctor. There are many causes of coughing apart from a chest infection, asthma being one of the more common, so it is important for the condition to be diagnosed correctly.

USUAL TREATMENT

Treatment depends on the type of chest infection. In the case of the overwhelming majority of chest infections, the cause is a viral infection and antibiotics may not help, although they are important in the treatment of bronchiectasis and secondary chest infections which may have spread to the lungs as a result of an infection somewhere else in the body.

While mild symptoms will respond to simple measures like humidifying the air with steam, severe bronchiolitis is likely to need hospital admission where the baby will be treated with oxygen and humidification, and possibly antibiotics if there is thought to be secondary infection. If your child is coughing up yellow or green sputum, or phlegm, this does not automatically mean that antibiotics are going to be helpful, but you should still have your child assessed by the doctor. If your doctor does prescribe antibiotics, these are likely to be a 'broad spectrum' antibiotic able to cope with a wide range of bacteria. The most

Chest Infections

USUAL TREATMENT *continued*

commonly prescribed drugs are amoxycillin and erythromycin.

There is little evidence that cough medicines are particularly helpful, but many parents buy and use them. As good as any is paediatric simple linctus BP, which you can buy from the chemist very cheaply. However, warm drinks and paracetamol are probably all that is needed. Cough suppressant medicines could well be harmful, since a cough can actually be a good thing: it is nature's way of clearing the chest, or preventing infection or irritation from reaching the chest. With small children and toddlers, persistent coughing may be soothed by a steamy atmosphere.

There is also a very clear link between adults who smoke and children who develop chest infections. If you must smoke, smoke outside. Avoid smoking in the car if your child is with you. Smoke irritates the lungs, and a child who has some other form of chest infection or irritation cannot possibly be helped by inhaling tobacco smoke produced by other people in the house.

Chickenpox

See also Shingles

Chickenpox is a common infectious illness, caused by the same virus that causes shingles.

SYMPTOMS

An itchy rash possibly accompanied by a temperature usually starts on the body as raised red spots (see pages 160–2 and illustration between pages 128 and 129), then spreads out to the legs, arms, head and face. These spots turn to blisters which crust over to form scabs. Children are infectious from five to six days before the spots appear until all the spots have developed scabs – about five days. It may take two weeks for the spots to disappear.

ACTION

If you are sure of the diagnosis, there is no need to see a doctor. Keep your child off school for six days after the spots appear, to avoid spreading the infection. For children who have had recent chemotherapy or radiotherapy, chickenpox can be a very serious illness. In addition, if your child is taking steroids, an injection of immunoglobulin may be necessary to boost the body's immunity.

USUAL TREATMENT

Try to persuade your child not to scratch the spots or pick at the scabs as this can leave scars. Paracetamol will help the fever and calamine will help the itching. Only children with immunity problems need specific treatment. Since chickenpox is more serious in adults, it is better to get it out of the way in childhood.

Chilblains

An itchy, purple-red swelling which typically affects toes or fingers in cold weather. They are caused by excessive narrowing of the tiny blood vessels just under the surface of the skin.

SYMPTOMS

These painful swellings most often occur on fingers and toes, but can also appear on other parts of the body such as the buttocks. They are triggered in cold weather by changes in blood vessels which are unusually sensitive to the cold, and in particular to changes in temperature. Cold weather causes a drop in circulation and reduces the skin's supply of oxygen, causing itching.

ACTION

The condition can be painful but it is otherwise harmless and has no connection with any other problems with the circulation. If you are confident of the diagnosis, there is no need for your child to see a doctor. If you aren't sure what the cause of the swelling is, then see your doctor for advice.

USUAL TREATMENT

Keeping your child's hands and feet warm, using gloves and socks, is by far the most valuable treatment. Make sure these items do not constrict the blood supply. Talcum powder can ease any itching. There are no drug treatments that are of particular value in children.

Cleft Lip and Palate

See also Speech Problems

An abnormality of development of the lip and/or the palate (the roof of the mouth). These conditions are present at birth in approximately 1 in every 800 babies. The cause is not known.

SYMPTOMS

In these conditions the child is born with a cleft, or split, in the top lip, or the two sides of the palate are not fully joined together. The child can have just one of these conditions or both together. A cleft palate will make feeding more difficult. Some children with these conditions have problems with hearing and speech later on.

ACTION

These conditions should be diagnosed immediately after birth, and will be treated by a team of hospital specialists.

USUAL TREATMENT

A cleft lip can be repaired surgically very soon after birth for cosmetic reasons, although some surgeons believe that better results are obtained if surgery is delayed for about three months. The cleft palate is also repaired surgically, usually at the age of approximately 12 months. If feeding is a problem with a cleft palate, special teats may be provided to ease this. Breast-feeding is frequently successful in the case of a cleft lip. For the great majority of children with these conditions, the skills of the surgeons mean that nowadays very little trace of the abnormality will be visible after treatment.

Clotting Disorders

See also Bruising ● Meningitis

When a blood vessel is damaged, special cells called platelets clump together at the site of the injury and react with chemicals known as clotting factors to stop bleeding. Insufficient platelets and low levels of clotting factors mean bleeding continues. The most common clotting disorder in children is called ITP (idiopathic thrombocytopenic purpura). Inherited genetic disorders include haemophilia, Christmas disease and von Willebrand's disease.

SYMPTOMS

Children with ITP may be perfectly healthy, but have low levels of platelets in the blood. The exact cause of ITP is unknown, but it is thought to follow a viral infection. Symptoms of clotting disorders include more bruising than expected for the level of injury, heavy nosebleeds, or blood in the urine or motions. In the case of haemophilia, your child may experience joint and muscle pain.

ACTION

If you suspect a clotting disorder, discuss it with your doctor who can make a full assessment and refer you to a specialist.

USUAL TREATMENT

While ITP usually gets better without treatment, some children may need admission to hospital and steroid drugs. Boys with haemophilia (girls may carry the disease but are not affected by it) will be given extra clotting factor.

Clumsiness

A wide-ranging term that covers the whole spectrum from the normal child who is just not quite as dextrous as others, to the child who has major difficulties with movement. A child with severe difficulties is usually referred to as having DCD (developmental co-ordination disorder).

SYMPTOMS

DCD can take many forms. It most often affects balance and co-ordination, fine and gross motor function, perception and sometimes speech. Fine motor function is the use of the hands, gross motor function refers to large body movements, and perception is the way that the brain interprets the world. Approximately 2 per cent of children can be classified as clumsy. While the more severe forms of clumsiness are quite often linked with learning problems, children with these difficulties have a wide range of levels of intelligence.

ACTION

If you are concerned about your child, consult your health visitor or doctor who may refer you for more detailed assessment either by a paediatrician, or by a paediatric physiotherapist or an occupational therapist.

USUAL TREATMENT

The great majority of children with clumsiness will develop into entirely normal adults. Their interests and expertise are perhaps more likely to develop in areas that don't require high levels of physical co-ordination. Children with more severe forms of DCD may need help in school and home to enable them to reach their full potential.

Coeliac Disease

A condition in which the child is sensitive to and therefore intolerant of foods containing gluten, a protein found in certain cereals such as wheat. The lining of the bowel appears to be damaged through this sensitivity, causing disappearance of the finger-like swellings known as villi which normally greatly increase the surface area of the bowel lining. Since there is so much less area for absorption, many nutrients fail to be absorbed by the digestive system.

SYMPTOMS

Children with coeliac disease may pass motions that are so fatty and greasy that they are almost impossible to flush away. This is caused by a failure of the body to absorb fat from the diet. Malabsorption has a number of consequences, including weight loss, poor appetite, slow development or anaemia. Other symptoms may include listlessness, a swollen abdomen, excess wind, diarrhoea or vomiting.

ACTION

Although fatty stools do not always mean coeliac disease, they should alert you to the possibility. Consult your doctor who may refer your child on to a paediatrician.

USUAL TREATMENT

Once the diagnosis has been confirmed by a doctor, the treatment is a gluten-free diet, and the doctor or a specialist dietitian will advise on this. Provided your child stays on this diet, the bowel should make a complete recovery and all symptoms should disappear. For more information, contact the Coeliac Society (see page 214) who can provide an invaluable range of information and advice.

Cold Sores

See also Impetigo

These are sores, caused by a virus, that typically occur around the mouth, especially on the edge of the lips and on the chin, and also on the nose or fingers.

SYMPTOMS

Cold sores look like tiny blisters, and are caused by the type 1 herpes simplex virus. This is completely different from the herpes virus that causes genital herpes. The first infection with the virus may cause a sore ulcerated mouth and possibly a fever. The virus then remains dormant in the skin, only to flare up as a sore if the child has a cold or other infection. These sores can also be triggered off by strong sunlight, stress or tiredness. Before the sores appear the skin tingles; they enlarge, become itchy, and then as they heal they crust over. The sore may become infected, in which case the blister becomes crusty, yellow and weeping.

ACTION

See the doctor to have the diagnosis confirmed and possibly for antiviral treatment. If the sore becomes infected, your child may be prescribed a course of antibiotic treatment. Cold sores are very infectious and your child will need his own towel and cup.

USUAL TREATMENT

Antiviral creams such as Zovirax can shorten the duration of the actual cold sore and speed up the healing process. As yet there are no treatments to prevent attacks happening altogether.

Colic

See also Intussusception ● Crying

Infantile colic is characterized by repeated episodes of inconsolable crying and even screaming in a baby aged under three months. The exact cause is not known but it is thought that the baby experiences abdominal pain, possibly caused by a spasm in the muscle that lines the colon (large intestine).

SYMPTOMS

During attacks the child is tense and rigid and cries or screams. Your baby may pull his or her knees up and the pains seem to come in sharp bursts, with lots of wind being passed after an attack. Between attacks your baby will seem quite well.

ACTION

All babies with colic should be checked over by a doctor at least once. The doctor may find nothing wrong, but this in itself can be reassuring. Pain that continues after 12 weeks of age is not colic and needs to be reassessed.

USUAL TREATMENT

Colic drops such as Infacol can be very helpful. Some herbal treatments, like fennel, can also help, but ask your health visitor's advice before using these. There is some evidence that cow's milk may make colic worse, so it might be worth using soya-based milks as a substitute for your normal baby milk if you are bottle-feeding. If you are breast-feeding, try reducing your own intake of dairy products, but talk to your health visitor first.

Colour Blindness

An inability to distinguish between various colours. Colour blindness is much more common in boys than in girls. About 8 per cent of all males and 1 per cent of females in Europe have some degree of colour blindness; the incidence is much lower in non-white races.

WHAT TO WATCH FOR

The most common form of colour blindness is an inability to distinguish between red and green. True colour blindness, in which no colours are distinguished at all, is extremely rare.

Colour blindness is sometimes only picked up during a routine school medical examination when your child is shown special colour charts. Alternatively, you or your child's teacher may notice that your child is consistently making errors choosing or identifying colours or shades. Children with colour blindness do not usually notice anything unusual themselves because, of course, they are unaware of the fact that other children see colours differently.

ACTION

If you suspect that your child may be colour-blind, consult your doctor who has special charts to help assess if this is the case.

USUAL TREATMENT

No treatment is needed, or even possible. However, recognizing the problem can be important for children, particularly when they start at school and may find that colour coding is used for marking property. If parents and teachers are aware of the problem, then they will be able to make suitable allowances.

Common Cold

A viral infection affecting the upper respiratory tract. On average, children tend to have seven colds a year.

SYMPTOMS

The main symptoms of a cold are a blocked or runny nose, streaming eyes, a sore throat and a slight fever. In small babies the airways in the nose are so small that they can easily become blocked, creating an alarming cacophony of snorting and snuffling, which thankfully is not usually as bad as it seems. Babies may find it difficult to feed if the nose is congested. Older children will also have learnt how to breathe through the mouth so colds never appear quite as dramatic with them.

ACTION

Colds usually last between five and seven days, though babies can stay snuffly for up to a week longer. For simple colds there is little point in seeing a doctor. However, there are occasions when you should seek medical help. These include a persistent fever of over 39°C (102°F) for more than 24 hours, or a fever less than this for three days or more. If your child also vomits, or seems unusually ill, if he or she has difficulty breathing or eating, or if he or she gets much worse after a few days, see your doctor.

USUAL TREATMENT

There is no cure for the common cold. Make sure your child is comfortable and encourage him or her to drink as much fluid as possible. Don't worry if your child isn't hungry. Nasal congestion can be helped by steam and using decongestant nose drops (never use them for more than five days). Paracetamol will help to lower the temperature and ease any discomfort. Secondary ear or chest infections might require antibiotic treatment.

Conjunctivitis

See also Foreign Bodies (in eye) ● Hayfever

Conjunctivitis is an irritation of the conjunctivae, the membranes that cover the front of the white of the eye and line the eyelids. The irritation can be caused by an allergic reaction or by an infection.

SYMPTOMS

In **allergic conjunctivitis** the conjunctivae may be red and itchy, but without the additional sticky yellow or creamy-coloured pus or gritty sensation that is seen in **infectious conjunctivitis**. Allergic conjunctivitis is frequently a symptom of hayfever or perennial rhinitis (the year-round version of hayfever) and may be associated with a runny or blocked nose.

Children with such allergies are often sufferers from either eczema or asthma, or may come from families with these problems. Infectious conjunctivitis is, as the name implies, very infectious and your child may have been in contact with someone with the condition. He or she may also have a cold or upper respiratory tract infection.

ACTION

If you think your child has an infection, gently wipe the eyes clean using cotton wool soaked in clean warm water. This is particularly soothing if there has been a build-up of discharge overnight. Unless the cause of conjunctivitis is very obvious – for instance, if redness comes on immediately following a swim –

then your child should always be assessed by a doctor. Consult a doctor right away if your child has a single red eye that isn't sticky, redness that develops after any form of eye injury, or if your child complains that his or her eyesight has suddenly become abnormal.

Conjunctivitis

USUAL TREATMENT

If your child has **allergic conjunctivitis** that is part of a wider picture of allergy, perhaps being associated with nasal symptoms, or has conditions such as asthma or eczema running in the family, then it may be most effectively treated with oral antihistamine medicines. Antihistamines such as Piriton (chlorpheniramine) are fairly sedative, but other drugs should not make your child sleepy. If antihistamine medications alone are not enough, or you or your doctor prefer to use a topical treatment (one that is used on the surface rather than being taken internally), then your child may be prescribed eye drops such as Opticrom (disodium cromoglycate). These are generally free of side-effects, but have to be used four times a day every day or for as long as the cause of the allergy is present. Many children eventually grow out of the condition.

Infectious conjunctivitis is usually treated with antibiotic drops or ointment. Without treatment, it is likely to persist for anything up to three weeks, but it will be cleared rapidly with the drops or ointments. These should usually be used until the condition is better, and then for a further 24 hours. Infectious conjunctivitis is highly contagious and can spread very easily around families, schools or playgroups. Scrupulous hygiene is essential. You should always use a separate flannel and towel for the affected child, and wash your hands carefully after using the eye drops or ointment. Children with infectious conjunctivitis should always be kept off school, playgroup or other communal activities until the condition has completely cleared up or at least until 48 hours after starting antibiotic treatment. This may seem an excessively strict restriction, especially if it means a parent has to stay off work to look after the child, but the condition is so infectious that this is an essential precaution.

Constipation

See also Anal Fissure ● Diet ● Soiling

Constipation occurs when your child has difficulty passing a bowel motion, and stools are hard and dry.

SYMPTOMS

Your child may seem reluctant to go to the toilet, and complain of pain or discomfort when he does.

ACTION

Children vary enormously in how often they pass a motion: it doesn't matter much how often your child goes if he or she is not in pain and passes a normal but infrequent motion. Breast-feeding often causes infrequent motions, but these are usually loose. Bottle-fed babies may develop constipation as a result of having a particular formula of milk. Any baby who has been unwell may become constipated as a result of reduced fluid intake and increased sweating.

USUAL TREATMENT

Babies may be helped by increased fluid intake, but never give babies or young children laxatives: they are rarely necessary, and may be harmful. Older children may lack fibre in their diet, so feed them fruit, baked beans, and cereals.

If your child seems continually constipated, then see your health visitor or doctor. Persistent severe constipation from birth may be caused by lack of thyroid hormone, or from a rare condition called Hirschsprung's disease in which part of the bowel wall does not contract normally because of a lack of nerve cells.

Convulsions

See also Epilepsy ● Fever

Convulsions, also known as fits or seizures, occur as a result of abnormal electrical activity in the brain, and may be caused by a high fever or conditions such as epilepsy.

SYMPTOMS

Convulsions typically produce abnormal movements, usually stiffness followed by shaking, twitching or jerking.

ACTION

The first time your child has a convulsion, call the doctor or an ambulance. If your child has a high temperature, it is vital to cool your child right down by stripping off clothing, gentle fanning or even tepid sponging. Do not try to give any medication by mouth during the convulsion. Lie your child on the floor on his or her side so that if he dribbles or vomits the liquid can drain out of the mouth and not be inhaled. Do not put anything in your child's mouth. Check for breathing after the fit has come to an end, but never start resuscitation during a convulsion. If your child has stopped breathing, call 999, then start emergency resuscitation (see page 93).

USUAL TREATMENT

It is essential that a child is thoroughly assessed after a first fit. This will probably be done at a hospital. There is no evidence that febrile convulsions in any way damage a child's intelligence. Only about one child in 50 who has febrile convulsions will develop epilepsy.

Cough

See also Asthma ● Chest Infections ● Croup

A cough is just a symptom, not an illness. Coughing is generally protective, and is nature's way of clearing the chest, or preventing infection or irritation from reaching the chest. For example, if you inhale a pea by mistake while eating a meal, the resulting cough shifts the pea and keeps it from becoming lodged in the airways. The cough that most people get when going into a smoke-filled room has a similar purpose.

SYMPTOMS

Every child coughs at times. There are different types of cough: a loose or phlegmy cough is usually caused by some form of infection; a dry cough may be the result of irritation, from fumes of smoke, for instance, or from the catarrh associated with a cold. A dry cough may be associated with asthma, especially if the cough seems to be worse at night or after exertion.

ACTION

Whether you consult a doctor depends on a number of factors, in particular your child's age. A cough in the first few weeks after birth can cause more problems than a cough later in life. Babies have tiny air passages and a relatively weak cough is not much use at expelling germs or other irritants from the airways.

With a baby, you should seek medical advice if :

● The cough lasts more than a couple of days

● The cough is associated with a raised temperature

● Your baby is off his or her food

● You are concerned that your baby seems in any other way to be unwell

In older children, you should see a doctor if:

Cough

ACTION *continued*

- Your child seems unwell
- Your child coughs mainly at night, or on exercising
- The cough started after an episode of choking (he or she may have inhaled a foreign body such as a peanut, bead or sweet)
- A cough persists after a cold

USUAL TREATMENT

The treatment of a cough will depend on the cause.

- Persistent croupy-type coughing may be soothed by a steamy atmosphere. Try taking the child into a shower room or bathroom, and leaving the hot water running (don't put the child under or into the hot water).

- For non-croupy coughs in the toddler and older child, warm drinks can be very soothing.

- If your doctor diagnoses a chest infection, then antibiotics may be needed. If the underlying cause is asthma, your doctor is likely to prescribe inhaled medication.

- If the cough is just a simple tickle with no underlying cause, there may be a case for using a mild cough medicine. The best, and the cheapest, is 'simple linctus BP'. This causes very few side-effects and can soothe an irritating tickle. If you require a more powerful cough-suppressing linctus, then try pholcodine linctus. Ask your doctor or pharmacist about the safe dose for your child's age.

Cradle Cap

See also Eczema

A harmless form of severe dandruff causing thickened and crusty patches on the scalp. This scaly appearance is typical of a condition known as seborrhoeic dermatitis. Cradle cap is most common in babies but can occur up to the age of six years.

SYMPTOMS

The appearance of cradle cap is of oily yellowish scales and patches on the scalp. Either small or large areas of the scalp may be affected. It can be associated with patches of dry scaly skin on the face, behind the ears and almost anywhere else on the body, even extending to the nappy area.

ACTION

Loosen the scales on the scalp at night with baby oil or even olive oil, then use a gentle shampoo the next day. Do not use medicated shampoo on small babies. See your doctor or health visitor if the condition does not improve or if it worsens.

USUAL TREATMENT

If the simple treatments described above don't work, your GP may recommend an emollient to soften the scales and the skin. If the scales are thick, your doctor may prescribe a mild steroid cream or lotion. Older children may need an anti-dandruff shampoo or possibly a mixture containing sulphur and salicylic acid to break down the crusts. The scalp may sometimes become infected and this could possibly need antibiotic treatment. If there are signs of eczema elsewhere on your child's body, then seek your doctor's advice.

Crawling – the child who doesn't...

See also Cerebral Palsy • Clumsiness

Most children start to crawl at around 8 to 10 months of age, but this is an average. Some will crawl sooner, and others later.

WHAT TO WATCH FOR

If your child is making no attempt to crawl or move around by 10 months, then talk to your health visitor. While there is a considerable natural variation between children in what is normal – some never crawl and go straight to walking, while others bottom-shuffle – they usually have to be able to get into the crawling position to be able to pull up to stand.

ACTION

While it is vitally important that children are laid on their backs when it is time for them to sleep (see Sudden Infant Death Syndrome, page 188), it is also important that they are laid on their tummies to play. This will encourage them to push up on their arms, strengthen their backs and necks, and facilitates getting into the crawling position. Children who are only ever laid on their backs may be put at a disadvantage unless they are very adventurous and roll over for themselves – which they should be able to do by about the age of six months.

USUAL TREATMENT

Your health visitor will advise you on activities to encourage your child's movement, and will refer you to a doctor for a more detailed assessment if she thinks there is a problem.

Croup

See also Chest Infections ● Cough

Croup is a barking cough and affects children under the age of three. It is caused by inflammation of the throat and upper airways following a respiratory infection.

SYMPTOMS

Croup starts remarkably suddenly, usually in the middle of the night. The child may have had a cold before the symptoms start. The noise of croup sounds like a cross between a seal barking and a child choking. Breathing is also noisy and difficult.

ACTION

Croup needs immediate treatment, ideally by inhaling steam. Take your child into the bathroom and leave the hot tap running (but keep your child away from direct contact with the water). Call a doctor if your child seems to be getting worse, or if home treatment is having no effect in 30 to 40 minutes. Never give cough medicines to a child with croup.

USUAL TREATMENT

Most cases of croup get better without specific treatment, but if the symptoms are severe enough your doctor may suggest using a nebulizer. This is a device that creates a fine mist of moisture usually containing budesonide (a form of steroid). Budesonide may be given by your doctor either before, or instead of, admission to hospital in less severe cases. About one in every ten children with croup is admitted to hospital, and, of these, 1 in 20 needs medical intervention to keep the airways clear.

Crying

All babies cry, for many reasons – it is almost their only means of communication. New parents automatically assume that the tears mean that their child is in deep distress, but this isn't necessarily the case.

WHAT TO WATCH FOR

Most crying occurs during the first 12 weeks of life. At six weeks, a quarter of babies will be crying or miserable for more than three hours a day. At three months of age, two hours of crying a day is typical, and more than three hours each day is common. This improves as the child gets older. Persistently crying babies are a real problem for parents. Some babies are very placid, while others cry all the time. The amount that they cry varies as much as the amount some adults talk. The parents of a crying baby often feel guilty, believing that if their baby continues to cry, then they must be doing something wrong. But if all babies cry, it is perfectly possible that the worst criers are just at one end of the normal spectrum. While this can be reassuring, it is important to try and find out why your child is crying, but do realize that you may not discover why.

ACTION

Check to see if your child is hungry or uncomfortable. If your baby seems unwell and has a cry that sounds different to his or her normal cry, then you should consult a doctor without delay. Sudden-onset crying in babies who don't usually cry also needs to be assessed, unless the cause is immediately obvious to you. Talk to your health visitor who can be a very good source of advice and guidance with crying children.

Crying

WHAT YOU CAN DO

This obviously depends on the cause of the crying. However, if you can't pinpoint what is going on, your doctor has checked your child over, and you have a persistently crying baby, then try the following:

● Pick your child up and carry him or her around as much as you can; babies seem to find the body contact soothing. Using a papoose or baby sling can be a simple way of doing this.

● Movement seems to calm many crying babies. This may involve walking up and down pushing the pram, or even driving your child round and round in the car.

● If, despite all your best efforts, the crying goes on and on and you feel yourself becoming increasingly desperate, then ask a friend or relative to help if this is at all possible. The combination of frustration, worry and exhaustion can be very stressful and someone else may be able to give you the brief breather that you so desperately need. The excellent self-help group Serene (incorporating the Cry-Sis helpline) has a team of volunteers who offer telephone support and who can be a real source of strength to desperate parents (see page 214).

● If it is absolutely impossible for you to get anyone to help and you are on your own and at the end of your tether with your crying and screaming baby, then put him down somewhere safe. Now leave the room for 10 minutes. Your baby won't come to any harm over this time. Try to cool down. Take a breath of fresh air. Have a cup of tea or coffee and try some slow, controlled, deep breathing. When you feel you have calmed down, return to your baby.

Cystic Fibrosis

A hereditary disease that prevents nutrients in food from being properly absorbed, affecting 1 in 2,500 children.

SYMPTOMS

Most children with this disease show signs of poor growth and have frequent chest infections. Poor growth results from sticky secretions in the pancreas which prevent the release of certain enzymes needed for digestion. There is excessive salt in the sweat, and the child has more frequent chest infections than average, and eventually a frequent productive cough, with thick yellow or green sputum. Sometimes there may be pale, oily motions. In some babies the bowel becomes blocked immediately after birth with abnormal faeces. This condition is called meconium ileus and often babies suffer from vomiting, a distended abdomen and constipation.

ACTION

Most cases are detected soon after birth. If you suspect that your child might have cystic fibrosis, consult your doctor right away. Your GP may refer your child to a paediatrician for detailed assessment and tests.

USUAL TREATMENT

Treatment usually includes pancreatic enzyme supplements, regular chest physiotherapy and antibiotics. A high-calorie diet is needed because the child is not able to absorb all the food eaten and also because energy requirements are 30 to 40 per cent higher than for other children. Vitamin supplements will also be part of the treatment. Try to get as much information about the condition as you can – the Cystic Fibrosis Trust (see page 214) is particularly helpful.

Deafness

See also Ear Problems

Any loss of hearing is described as deafness. Happily, most childhood deafness is temporary, but as it can nevertheless still have a profound effect at a critical time for learning it must be taken seriously. There are two main types of deafness:

CONDUCTIVE DEAFNESS
In this condition the conduction of sound through the ear is obstructed. This can be due to a blockage in the outer ear canal, usually with wax. A certain amount of earwax is healthy – it protects the delicate skin in the ear canal from irritation and inflammation. Normally the body removes it to the outer part of the ear where it can be gently wiped away. However, if it builds up inside the ear, it can cause an obstruction and sometimes pain and deafness. The blockage can also be in the middle ear cavity and can be caused by glue ear, a type of middle ear infection, in which the fluid in the middle ear cavity is thick and sticky. Rarely, conductive deafness is caused by damage to the eardrum due to sudden changes of pressure in an aircraft, or to a perforated eardrum after an injury.

NERVE DEAFNESS
In this type of deafness the hearing problem lies in the inner ear itself, either in the nerve that sends impulses from the ear to the brain, or within the brain. This form of deafness is most typically present from birth, when it can be the result of conditions such as rubella contracted by the mother before the baby's birth. It can also be caused by meningitis, severe jaundice occurring shortly after birth and a few other causes, such as a severe shortage of oxygen at birth.

SYMPTOMS

If your child does not hear when you say something – particularly if it is a pleasant word such as 'sweets' – then there is likely to be a problem with hearing. An older child may be able to tell you about any difficulty, but it is more likely that you may get a clue if a child is always shouting, or if the television set is turned up loudly. With younger children, the main clue is a delay in learning to speak, or even lack of clarity in speech. Watch for these clues:

● Your baby is six months old and does not respond consistently to sound.

● Your child is one year old and has either not started babbling, or else has started but then stopped.

● Your toddler speaks no words.

● Your two-year-old does not make two-word phrases.

● Your two-and-a-half-year-old has speech that is not generally intelligible to you or the family.

● Your three-year-old is not making sentences.

ACTION

Routine hearing checks are performed on all babies but, in addition, watch for any possible hearing problems or difficulties with speech. If you are in any doubt about your child's ability to hear, then seek advice.

Most earwax will clear automatically. If you see any in the outer part of your child's ear and want to remove it, simply use a cotton bud to wipe it away gently. Never insert the bud into the ear canal as this will push the wax further into the ear, making it likely to become compacted inside. This will make the wax even harder, and it may need to be removed by syringing. As a simple rule, never insert anything smaller than your elbow into the ear canal. This might sound absurd, but it is essential.

Deafness

USUAL TREATMENT

The treatment of deafness depends on what exactly the diagnosis is. The sooner the diagnosis is made, and treatment is started, the better.

CONDUCTIVE DEAFNESS

The aim of the treatment is to eliminate whatever is causing the blockage of transmission of sound into the ear.

Wax is easily loosened and removed by using sodium bicarbonate or olive oil drops, followed if necessary by gentle syringing by the doctor or nurse. Glue ear can be treated in a number ways, including the insertion of grommets by an ENT (ear, nose and throat) surgeon, but many cases of glue ear will recover without treatment. Grommets are tiny plastic tubes that are inserted, under an anaesthetic, through a slit made in the ear drum. These allow air to pass into the middle ear cavity, and this allows the pressure in the middle ear cavity to return back to normal and be equal with the pressure of the air outside. Recently, some doctors have begun to question whether this operation is essential, though sometimes it can be remarkably effective.

NERVE DEAFNESS

It may be necessary to use a hearing aid to improve nerve deafness. As a parent you may feel upset or disappointed that your child has to use an aid, but the quicker you can help your child adapt to using the aid, the better. With severe hearing difficulties it would be sensible and a good long-term investment if you have special training in lip reading or signing.

Dehydration

See also Diarrhoea ● Vomiting

A condition that results from a shortage of fluid in the body, typically as a result of sickness and diarrhoea.

SYMPTOMS

The younger the child, the more at risk he or she is of becoming dehydrated. Watch for these signs:

- Watery diarrhoea
- Very dry mouth
- Unable to keep down fluids without vomiting

- Not passing urine for 6 hours
- Listlessness, tiredness, sleepiness
- Pale colour
- Sunken eyes
- Baby's sunken fontanelle

ACTION

If your child appears to be significantly dehydrated then contact you doctor now. Severe dehydration can be very serious, even fatal and your child may need to be admitted to hospital and given fluids through a drip.

USUAL TREATMENT

If your child has diarrhoea and vomiting, do what you can to prevent dehydration by giving as much fluid as your child will take. Children who are reluctant to drink or eat or who have profuse diarrhoea should be given prescribed mixtures of dextrose and electrolytes. Water tends not to be very well absorbed if given by itself.

Depression

See also Sleep Problems

Depression is a medical condition as well as the general feeling of being 'down'.

SYMPTOMS

In the under-fives, the chief symptoms are tearfulness and unhappiness, sleep disturbance, difficulty concentrating and sometimes being excessively argumentative with bad behaviour. If your child seems constantly unhappy for no very obvious reason, cries frequently for no obvious reason and seems very lethargic, then depression should be considered.

ACTION

Talk to your child. There might be a very simple explanation for the feelings, perhaps a fear that you haven't recognized or a misunderstanding that frightens the child. However, if you can't get to the bottom of the problem, go to see your doctor.

USUAL TREATMENT

The doctor will perform an examination to rule out any underlying physical cause that could be affecting mood or energy, or refer your child for assessment by a child psychologist or psychiatrist, often at a family centre. The family centre teams have great expertise at dealing with childhood depression and will spend time talking to your child to unravel the cause of the problem. They can advise on treatment or medication. Treatment will very much depend on the causes and the individual problem. The majority of children make an excellent recovery.

Diabetes

An excessive build-up of sugar in the blood. This is caused by a shortage of the hormone insulin which is produced by the pancreas and controls the absorption of sugar.

SYMPTOMS

Children tend to develop diabetes quickly. Typical symptoms are:

- Excessive thirst
- Tiredness
- Frequent passing of urine
- Weight loss
- Irritability
- Smelly breath

ACTION

If your child has symptoms of diabetes, see a doctor quickly. If possible, take a sample of your child's urine with you. Untreated diabetes can result in a coma, and, in rare circumstances, even death.

USUAL TREATMENT

The doctor will test your child's urine, and if sugar is present, will probably arrange an immediate assessment by a hospital paediatrician. The mainstay of treatment is to replace insulin by injection since it is destroyed in the stomach if given by mouth. You will also be seen by a dietician who will explain how important it is for your child to eat a healthy diet.

Diarrhoea

See also Coeliac Disease ● Dehydration
● Gastroenteritis ● Intussusception ● Vomiting

Frequent, watery stools often accompanied by vomiting.

SYMPTOMS

It is the *change* in pattern and consistency of motions that is important to note. Breast-fed infants may have half a dozen fairly loose stools every day but this does not mean that they have diarrhoea. The most common cause of watery diarrhoea is gastroenteritis, when it is often accompanied by vomiting. Other infections occurring elsewhere in the body can also cause diarrhoea, especially in small children. Your child may also have abdominal pain and a fever.

Some children seem to be sensitive to particular foods or to a change in water, and excessive drinking of fruit juices and sugary liquids might produce diarrhoea, as may weaning foods such as apple purée or mashed banana. There is a small but definite group of children, usually aged between six months and two years, who have persistent diarrhoea but are otherwise perfectly well. Provided they are fit and otherwise healthy and are growing normally, such children are not a cause for concern.

ACTION

The single most important reason for seeking urgent medical attention for your child is dehydration (see page 71). You should also always contact a doctor if your child has bloody diarrhoea. The most likely cause may be infection, but your doctor will want to exclude rarer conditions such as intussusception (see page 136). If diarrhoea and vomiting continue for more than 24 hours, contact your doctor.

Diarrhoea

USUAL TREATMENT

In treating acute diarrhoea, the first thing to do is to prevent the chief hazard, dehydration. Fluids are essential. A child with a fever requires even more fluid. Fluid replacement is the mainstay of the treatment of gastroenteritis. Children with profuse diarrhoea should be given special mixtures that contain dextrose and electrolytes. These are sold under trade names such as Dioralyte or Rehidrat. These sachets should be mixed with the specified amounts of water. Antibiotics may make many forms of diarrhoea worse, and starvation makes little or no difference. Drugs such as kaolin are little help, and more powerful drugs such as Lomotil may even be dangerous. They work by slowing down the bowel and stop the diarrhoea leaving the system. However, they have no effect on preventing the fluid from accumulating in the intestine.

Giving your child drugs like this may make you feel better – in that your child's diarrhoea may seem to stop – but they are not really doing any good. Your child is still losing water and salts into the intestine, but you won't know about it and can feel falsely reassured. This type of drug can also stop the viruses or bacteria from being expelled from the bowel, and can have seriously dangerous side-effects, even leading to severe muscle spasms.

If the diarrhoea continues for more than four or five days, then your doctor might ask you to collect a small sample of motion for analysis in the laboratory. Occasionally diarrhoea is caused by bacteria that can be helped by antibiotics. A bacteria known as campylobacter, which can be caught from pets and poor hygiene in food preparation, can cause diarrhoea and is easily dealt with by the antibiotic erythromycin. However, since antibiotics will make many forms of diarrhoea worse, doctors will want to know exactly which bacteria they are dealing with, rather than guessing – hence the need for a specimen.

Diarrhoea that continues despite all the treatment and advice detailed here will certainly need investigating. In babies this might be caused by coeliac disease, or even possibly by cystic fibrosis.

Diet

See also Abdominal Pain ● Diarrhoea ● Growth
Disorders ● Vomiting

Diet refers to the food eaten by your child. It should contain a
good balance of the main food groups (carbohydrate, protein
and fat). It is also important that older children have sufficient
fibre and avoid excess salt and sugar. If your child is eating a
mixed diet, he or she will probably be getting enough essential
vitamins and minerals for healthy growth.

COMMON WORRIES

FUSSY EATERS

Food fads and refusing to eat are
the commonest feeding problems
in young children – particularly
toddlers who would often rather
play than eat – causing parents
no end of worry. Fads may take
the form of always wanting to eat
exactly the same foods or being
excessively fussy about food.

WEIGHT GAIN

One of the greatest areas of concern
to parents is their child's growth –
and whether they're putting on too
much or too little weight.

In a baby, weight gain is often
seen as an indicator of how well
he is developing. However, since
birthweights vary enormously,
health professionals measure
growth on a specially devised
chart using a system of 'centile
lines'. This means a baby's
growth can be monitored on an
individual basis. Although
parents of hungry babies worry
they might be putting on too
much weight, the latest research
suggests that there is no link
between large babies and obese
adults. It's also practically
impossible to overfeed a baby.
They have very good appetite
mechanisms and generally will
not eat more than they require.

While too many sugary
snacks are to be discouraged,
children under two still require a
calorie-rich diet, which includes
full-fat dairy products and a
medium amount of fibre. Young
children should never be put on
a low-calorie or low-fat diet.

ACTION

FUSSY EATERS

If your child seems to be very faddy, and you are concerned that he or she is missing vital nutrients, then your health visitor should be able to give you advice about how to deal with this. However, do not take too narrow a view of your child's diet. Taken over a single day, the quality may seem to be poor, especially if your child is going through a faddy stage, but taken over a matter of weeks, the quality of the diet may well average out to be far more acceptable than you realize. Try to make sure that your child is having enough calcium (usually by drinking milk) and avoid giving him or her foods that are high in sugar.

Almost all feeding problems can be considered to be behavioural rather than happening because the child is unwell. Parental anxiety, although understandable, can worsen the situation significantly. When you find yourself worrying about your child's eating, the first and most important step is to *work out exactly what your worries are*. This may sound obvious: you're worried because your child doesn't eat. But you need to know just what it is about the pattern of not eating that concerns you so much.

Start by checking two things. Firstly, have your child properly weighed and measured, and have these results plotted on a chart. You can do this yourself, or your doctor or health visitor can do it for you. If you see that growth is entirely normal, then you can begin to relax about nutrition.

Secondly, you must find out exactly what your child really is eating. For instance, if you are worried that your child doesn't seem hungry, he or she could be eating more snacks between meals than you realize. The simplest way to monitor exactly what is eaten is to keep a food diary. Record everything that your child eats over a fortnight. Any one day may show an apparently dreadful diet, but averaged out you may be surprised how good your child's nutrition really is.

Discipline is also a major cause of concern at mealtimes. Discipline is obviously important, but it makes sense to take notice of the experience of countless parents over the years that battles will get you nowhere. It is very easy for parents to nag their child so much to 'eat it up' at mealtimes

Diet

that the anxiety that is created makes the situation worse. A child who is tense at mealtimes will be less likely to eat enough for his or her needs, and will therefore be more likely to ask for snacks between meals.

WEIGHT GAIN
- Try not to be too anxious about your baby's weight. It will be closely monitored by the clinic in the early months anyway. At this stage it is regularity of weight gain that matters – not weekly fluctuations.

- If you are concerned about your toddler or pre-school child's weight, ask your health visitor to plot his or her height and weight on a centile chart. Children vary so much in size that it is impossible to give a simple estimate of desirable weight at a particular age. Instead, the weight and height need to be compared.

SOLUTIONS

FUSSY EATERS

If you are concerned that your child's diet may be lacking certain nutrients, then vitamin supplements may help, but talk to your doctor or health visitor before starting on these and do not exceed the recommended dose. Too much can be as harmful as too little. If you have a child with a medical condition that requires special diets (coeliac disease or diabetes, for example) ask your doctor to refer you to a specialist dietitian for advice.

If your child seems to refuse everything put in front of her, try to follow these simple hints:

- Decide what you are worried about – when you have pinpointed your real concern and examined it, it will be more easy to deal with it.

- Serve less than your child will eat, not more.

- Don't rush or nag your child at mealtimes.

- Try to keep meals to a regular routine.

Diet

SOLUTIONS *continued*

- Don't worry about the order in which your child eats his or her courses.

- Don't serve food you know he or she doesn't like.

- Avoid giving too many drinks at mealtimes – there may not be room left for food.

- Try to make mealtimes fun.

If your child seems in any way unwell, or if repeated vomiting or abdominal pain is linked with the refusal to eat, you should consult your doctor. In addition, consult your doctor or health visitor if you are concerned about your child's growth.

WEIGHT GAIN

If there are concerns, your health visitor will be able to offer dietary advice and regular re-weighing.

- With babies, always make up the feeds using the right amount of formula. Dilute fruit juice with plenty of water.

- Don't put your toddler or older child on a diet, instead change it to include more unrefined foods, such as wholemeal bread, fresh fruit and vegetables. Cut down on sweets, biscuits and sugary drinks.

- Encourage your child to be as active as possible.

Down's Syndrome

This is a chromosomal abnormality present from conception. It is the most common congenital cause of severe learning difficulties. The incidence of Down's syndrome in liveborn babies is about 1 in 650, but the chance of having a baby with Down's syndrome becomes much greater the older the mother. For this reason, many women over the age of 35 or younger women with a history of Down's syndrome in the family are usually offered an amniocentesis test at around 16 weeks of pregnancy to check for Down's syndrome.

SYMPTOMS

Down's syndrome is usually diagnosed at, or shortly after, birth. Typical physical characteristics are a round face, abnormal skin creases on the palms and soles, protruding tongue and small ears. Heart problems are common. The diagnosis must be confirmed by chromosome analysis.

ACTION

Parents with a baby with Down's syndrome should receive a great deal of advice, support and counselling both at the time of diagnosis and in the ensuing months and years. It is a good idea to get in touch with other parents with children with this condition, to exchange ideas, opinions, stories, suggestions and problems.

USUAL TREATMENT

There is no treatment for this condition, and Down's syndrome children will usually have special educational needs. Heart checks and possibly surgery may be needed. All parents who have had a Down's syndrome baby will be offered specialist counselling to look into their particular risk.

Earache

See also Antibiotics ● Deafness

Pain in the ear is very common in the first five years. Earache can have many causes, including various types of ear infection, congestion of the eustachian tube (the tube that connects the middle ear to the back of the nose), throat infections (in which the pain is felt in the ear) and even teething. Infections most commonly occur in either the middle ear (otitis media) or the outer ear (otitis externa). Pain can also be felt in the ear during a flight.

OTITIS MEDIA (MIDDLE EAR INFECTION)
There is a one in three chance of a child having an episode of otitis media by the age of three years, and many children have repeated infections. Infections are most common between six months and two to three years, but very occasionally cause problems up to the teenage years. Infections enter the middle ear cavity from the throat through the eustachian tube, *not* from the outer part of the ear.

OTITIS EXTERNA (OUTER EAR INFECTION)
Otitis externa is less common in young children but can still cause problems. Anything that scratches the very delicate skin lining the outer part of the ear up to the ear drum can trigger this condition. The most common culprits are cotton buds, so never push these into the ear canal. The other major aggravating factor can be swimming. Water getting into the ear from swimming pools, which may not always be completely clean, can lead to sogginess, inflammation and infection of the skin of the ear canal.

Earache

PROBLEMS WHEN FLYING

The change in air pressure during take-off and landing often causes a very uncomfortable earache in both children and adults. Usually air can travel down the eustachian tube and out into the nose or mouth to equalize the pressure, but if there is any obstruction (e.g., from a cold), then pain is felt.

SYMPTOMS

Older children are able to tell you if their ear is painful, but for babies it can be much harder to diagnose. Symptoms can include crying, screaming, being generally and vaguely unwell, having a fever, and even loose motions or vomiting. Many parents come to recognize the cry of a child with earache. It is often a high-pitched wailing that sounds quite different from other cries.

the pain. When this happens the outer ear fills up with discharge, and pus and even blood may appear in the ear canal. Perforations usually heal leaving no damage, but your doctor should check the ear drum a week or so after such a perforation. Infections that do not clear completely, or perforations that do not heal, can cause deafness.

OTITIS MEDIA

Most middle-ear infections follow a cold or sore throat. As the infection builds up, the lining of the eustachian tube swells, in the same way that your nose becomes blocked when you have a cold. The pus in the middle ear cavity cannot drain away, and this leads to pressure on the ear drum which causes pain. Sometimes the pressure builds up so greatly that the ear drum perforates or bursts, which instantly relieves

OTITIS EXTERNA

The main symptoms of otitis externa are earache, sometimes itching, and discharge from the ear. The pain resulting from this type of infection tends to be different from that of otitis media, and it usually hurts if you tug gently on the ear. The area around the ear can sometimes be slightly tender. The opening of the ear canal may well be swollen, and there is likely to be a greeny, white or yellow discharge.

Earache

SYMPTOMS *continued*

PROBLEMS WHEN FLYING
If your child has a cold or catarrh, and there is any obstruction to air flowing along the eustachian tube, the ear drum bulges in (if you are landing), or out (if you are taking off), and this causes pain. In rare cases, these problems cause temporary deafness.

ACTION

There are a number of circumstances in which you should consult a doctor **immediately** with a child with earache. These are:

- If your child has a stiff neck (see also Meningitis, page 146)

- If your child banged his or her head shortly before the earache started

- Your child walks or stands unsteadily or seems to act 'drunk'

- If your child seems very ill and has a high fever

OTITIS MEDIA AND OTITIS EXTERNA
In the case of a suspected ear infection in babies over 7kg in weight, give paracetamol or ibuprofen. In addition, lots of cuddles and sympathy will always be welcome. The pain can also be eased by a warm flannel or hot water bottle held against the ear, but make sure that these are not too hot. If the pain does not settle with these measures, consult your doctor.

PROBLEMS WITH FLYING
As in adults, repeated swallowing helps keep the pressures in the ear equal. For this reason you should give your child a drink on take-off or landing and during the last 20 minutes or so of the flight. If your child's ears don't clear by swallowing, they will clear automatically if he or she cries, so if babies want to cry at this stage, let them.

Earache

USUAL TREATMENT

The doctor will examine your child, looking in particular at the ear drums using an instrument called an otoscope, and will discuss with you whether antibiotics are likely to be helpful.

OTITIS MEDIA

Doctors are actually still somewhat undecided as to how important antibiotics are in treating otitis media. In the long term there is no evidence at all that they make much difference, but it is possible that pain is relieved slightly sooner if antibiotics are given early. However, these are almost certainly not essential, and paracetamol may be all that is needed.

Children under five will usually be given amoxycillin or erythromycin. Check with your doctor how long the course of treatment should be. If there has been a perforation of the ear drum, with pus in the outer ear, your doctor will need to check the ear drum after the infection has recovered.

OTITIS EXTERNA

Treatment will be either with antibiotic medicines or drops, or both. Otitis externa can be quite difficult to clear up. The blind-ended tube that forms this part of the ear is the perfect breeding ground for bacteria, so several courses of the prescribed treatment may be needed.

PROBLEMS WHEN FLYING

Even on the longest journeys it is unwise to give your child any form of sedative. They are rarely effective, and can make the child even more miserable than usual when she wakes. If she is congested, or has a cold, decongestant nose drops or spray given before the flight may prevent earache. Any pain or deafness that remains after the flight may be helped by nose drops and painkillers.

Eczema

See also Impetigo

A skin condition causing dry, inflamed and often itchy skin. Some children have a tendency to develop eczema because the disorder, as well as asthma or hayfever, runs in their family. This is known as 'atopic' eczema. Less commonly, there is a specific external trigger that causes the problem. This type of eczema may be known as 'contact dermatitis'. The words 'eczema' and 'dermatitis' are interchangeable.

SYMPTOMS

The mildest form of eczema is simply dry skin. If the eczema becomes more severe, the skin becomes drier and more inflamed, with cracking, redness, soreness and itching, or any combination of these. Eczema can start in infancy, where all the skin may feel dry and a rash may appear on the face, scalp, trunk and outside of the legs and the arms. Black or dark-skinned children may have areas of paler skin, particularly on the face. In older children the rash primarily affects the fronts of the elbows, the backs of the knees, the neck, the feet, wrists and the hands – though it may occur anywhere.

Eczema can be aggravated by many things, in particular soap, which has a drying effect on the skin. Wool or other fabrics may irritate some children. Sometimes something in the child's diet may make the condition worse, though probably only to a significant degree in about 1 child in 20. In the other 19, diet makes no difference, so be sure to consult your doctor before altering what your child eats.

ACTION

A child with eczema should initially be seen by a doctor to have the diagnosis confirmed, for advice on management and

Eczema

ACTION *continued*

treatment. If your child has already seen a doctor, he or she should return if the rash gets worse, in particular if any areas become redder or look more inflamed or infected, or if the rash seems to be spreading or has crusts or scabs. Learn as much as you can about the condition and consider joining a self-help group such as the National Eczema Society (see page 215).

USUAL TREATMENT

There is no cure for eczema. Treatment is aimed at keeping the signs and symptoms to a minimum. If you go to your doctor for the first time and receive treatment which successfully clears the rash, only to have it return when the treatment is discontinued, this does not mean that the treatment was unsuccessful. This is simply the nature of the problem. It is tedious to have to continue using treatments, but essential if you are going to minimize the effects of the condition.

Emollients, which soften and moisten the skin, are the mainstay of treatment, and are particularly helpful when added to the bath water. More severe eczema needs anti-inflammatory steroid creams. For most children these will only be necessary for a short while, and the benefits of using them greatly outweigh any disadvantages. In addition you should also:

- Watch out for things that may be aggravating your child's eczema, such as woollen clothes. Cotton is much better, and far less likely to be an irritant.

- Keep your child's fingernails short to prevent scratching if the skin itches.

- Consider dietary changes if nothing else seems to help, but talk to your doctor about this first.

The good news is that half of all affected children will be free of the condition by the age of six years and most will have grown out of it by the age of 10.

Elbow Injuries

See also Fractures

A pulled elbow is a very common injury in toddlers.

SYMPTOMS

This problem can occur when your child pulls against you when you are holding his or her hand, if you swing the child around by the arms, or if you suddenly pull on the arm. One of the bones in the elbow joint temporarily pulls out of place, and while it usually returns to normal straight away, one of the ligaments can be trapped between the bones and this leaves the child reluctant or unable to use the arm. Your child will probably hold the arm slightly bent, with the palm facing downwards.

ACTION

If your child cannot move the arm, then do consult a doctor right away. Go to an accident and emergency unit, unless you live in a rural area where it might be worth phoning your doctor's surgery for advice first.

USUAL TREATMENT

Every doctor is taught a simple manoeuvre that will 'un-pull' the elbow quickly and relatively painlessly, so do seek help right away. Occasionally the joint sorts itself out as you are on your way to the hospital, and you arrive there to find your child is happy, healthy and painfree – a recipe for embarrassment and relief for parents. Don't ignore the problem, however, as it can be very painful for the child until it has been sorted out – always have the elbow checked as a precaution.

Epilepsy

See also Convulsions

Epilepsy is diagnosed when repeated convulsions, or seizures, occur over a period of months or years.

SYMPTOMS

Epileptic convulsions are typically caused by a burst of abnormal electrical impulses in the brain. There are two main types of seizure: 'tonic-clonic seizures' (formerly called 'grand mal') and 'absence seizures' (or 'petit mal'). In a tonic-clonic seizure the child becomes unconscious, goes stiff, falls over and the limbs may shake uncontrollably. It may well be associated with tongue-biting and incontinence. The seizure is followed by a period of drowsiness, and probably no memory of what has happened. In absence seizures, the child suddenly stops what he or she is doing, looks vacant, appears to stare momentarily and then carries on with what he or she was doing. These seizures may occur without anyone noticing, or just thinking the child is day-dreaming.

ACTION

If your child has had a first fit (see Convulsions, page 59) talk to your doctor. A brain scan will be done to confirm the diagnosis.

USUAL TREATMENT

Your child will need to see a hospital specialist to start treatment with medication which has to be taken regularly to prevent seizures. Medication will normally be continued until your child has been free of fits for at least two years.

Fainting

See also Convulsions

An episode of unconsciousness caused by a temporary reduction of the blood supply to the brain.

SYMPTOMS

Fainting is usually caused by a sudden drop of blood pressure. Faints are usually due to a raised temperature, hunger, exertion, a hot room, upset or shock, or suddenly standing up from a sitting or crouching position. The fall in blood pressure means that insufficient blood reaches the brain, and fainting is nature's way of making the child lie down. Lying down brings the head to the same level as the heart and allows blood to reach the brain again. Just before the faint your child will be hot and sweaty and pale, and may complain of a buzzing sound in the ears and of black spots before the eyes. He may then collapse, become unconscious, but recover in a minute or two.

ACTION

If your child is able to sit down or lower the head between the knees, it is usually possible to stop the faint coming on. If your child has already fainted, raise his or her feet until they are slightly higher than the head. This allows more blood to reach the brain. If your child has repeated episodes of fainting, consult your doctor who may want to arrange investigations to make certain that this is not a type of convulsion.

USUAL TREATMENT

Fainting rarely requires treatment.

Fever

See also Convulsions

Having a fever simply means having a temperature above normal. Fever is a symptom, not an illness. It is almost always the result of an infection with either viruses or bacteria. A raised temperature is part of the body's normal response to such infection and is almost certainly part of the way in which the body attempts to fight off the offending organisms.

SYMPTOMS

A normal temperature is defined as being 37°C (98.4°F). Sometimes you will know that your child has a temperature because he or she is so hot, but at other times you may need to use a thermometer. Other symptoms of fever may include shivering or feeling cold, or sweating and feeling hot. Children with a very high fever feel ill and may even have a fit – known as a febrile convulsion. Infections are by far the major cause of raised temperatures, but occasionally a consistently slightly raised temperature can be a sign of some other inflammatory problem, such as arthritis or bowel inflammation.

ACTION

If your child seems very sick, then consult a doctor whatever the temperature. If your child has a temperature higher than 39.5°C (102.5°F), then seek medical advice, though significantly high temperatures are actually very common at the start of many childhood illnesses.

You should seek medical help immediately if a baby has a temperature of over 40°C (104°F). The single most important thing that you can do with a hot child is cool him down. That may sound ridiculously simple, but countless parents ignore it as they are often

Fever

ACTION *continued*

frightened that if they don't keep their child wrapped up, then he will get worse. There is no truth in this at all. Many parents who bring their child to the doctor's surgery are often embarrassed that the child is so much better when they arrive. It is likely that they feel better because the trip out to the surgery has cooled them down. I know that many parents are still very reluctant to take a child with a temperature out of the home to see the doctor, but in fact the journey usually does no harm at all.

If your child is hot, cool him or her down.

- Firstly, remove most of the child's clothes – possibly just leaving on a thin vest or nightie.

- If necessary, a cooling fan can be helpful, though this should not be aimed directly at the child.

- Tepid sponging or even giving a tepid bath can also help tremendously and be very soothing. As the water evaporates from your child's hot skin, it will cool the skin very effectively.

- Don't forget to give your child plenty of cool drinks.

USUAL TREATMENT

In treating fevers the most important and valuable type of medication is paracetamol. Aspirin is no longer considered safe in children aged under 12, and should never be given. The chief alternative to paracetamol is ibuprofen, an anti-inflammatory drug with brand names including Junifen, Brufen and Nurofen. Always choose a sugar-free form if you can. Paracetamol is remarkably free from side-effects, provided the dose is not exceeded, and ibuprofen is valuable and safe for most children though is not advised in children with asthma as it can sometimes make wheezing worse.

Fifth Disease

This is sometimes known as 'slapped cheek disease' because of the red rash produced on the cheeks. Its unusual name comes from the fact that it was the fifth of the common childhood rashes, after measles, rubella, chickenpox and scarlet fever.

SYMPTOMS

It usually affects children aged between 3 and 12 years and begins with a bright red rash on the cheeks, making the child look as if she has been firmly slapped (see illustration between pages 128 and 129). The skin around the mouth is not discoloured, and in mild cases the rash may be barely noticeable. A fine, lacy, spotty red rash then appears on the limbs and trunk, and will come and go over the next month, often getting worse on exercise, exposure to the sun or on getting hot.

ACTION

Since this is a viral infection there is no treatment. Children with this condition tend not to be ill, but you should seek advice if your child has sickle-cell anaemia. The virus can also affect an unborn foetus, so if your child has been in contact with someone who is pregnant, make sure you tell the expectant mum to talk to her doctor and midwife. Your child is infectious before the rash appears but probably not once it is visible.

USUAL TREATMENT

Fifth disease usually needs no treatment. Your child is not infectious after the rash appears. Despite this, many school medical authorities advise that children should remain off school until the rash has disappeared.

If you ever have to call 999, you will be asked whether you want the fire, police, or ambulance service. For any of the emergencies detailed here, ask for the ambulance service.

You may hear the operator tell the ambulance station the phone number you are calling from. They know this automatically for most types of phone.

You will be asked for your address, or where the casualty is. If you are outside or in the car, do try to be precise. Give a road name if you know it, or some other landmark to help the crew find you. But don't panic if you don't know. As long as you are not using a mobile phone, the crew will be able to trace your position from the phone number. Give simple details of what has happened, who you are, and any other information that could be helpful – traffic hazards, for instance.

THE ABC OF RESUSCITATION
What to do first

Before rushing to help an injured child, first check there is no further danger. Don't move an injured child unless necessary. Shout for help and get someone to call an ambulance. Check if the child is conscious by gently squeezing his shoulders or calling his name. If a child is unconscious, follow the ABC of resuscitation:

A IS FOR AIRWAY
Ensure the airway is clear so oxygen can reach the brain.

Remove any obstruction in the mouth; put two fingers under the child's chin (one finger for a baby under 12 months) and one hand on his forehead, then tilt the head back gently.

B IS FOR BREATHING
Spend 10 seconds checking breathing. Is the chest rising and falling? Feel for breath against your cheek. If he's breathing, put him in the recovery position (see illustrations between pages 96 and 97); if he isn't breathing, but

First Aid

has a pulse, you will have to breathe for him by giving mouth-to-mouth ventilation till help arrives (see illustrations between pages 96 and 97).

C IS FOR CIRCULATION
The blood must circulate to carry oxygen to the brain. If the heart stops and there's no pulse, giving chest compressions will drive the blood through the heart and round the body. It must be done together with mouth-to-mouth ventilation, called CPR – cardiopulmonary resuscitation (see illustrations). To check for a pulse, feel for the large muscle at the side of the neck or, with a baby, the upper arm.

What to do if a child is unconscious, but breathing and has a pulse

FOR A CHILD
Put her in the recovery position (see illustrations between pages 96 and 97) to ensure she doesn't inhale vomit.

FOR A BABY
Hold him in your arms on one side, with his head down (see illustrations).

What to do if a child isn't breathing, but has a pulse

Give mouth-to mouth ventilation. To do this:

- Clear any obstruction from his mouth, tilt his head back.

- Pinch the nostrils closed and seal your mouth around his open mouth (see illustrations between pages 96 and 97) – round the lips and nose of a baby.

- Breathe into the child's lungs so his chest rises.

- Remove your mouth and let the chest fall, keeping the nostrils pinched.

- Continue for one minute (about 20 breaths).

- Call for an ambulance and continue giving mouth-to-mouth ventilation until help arrives.

What to do if a child isn't breathing and there is no pulse

You must start CPR – cardio-pulmonary resuscitation – which is a combination of chest

THE ABC OF RESUSCITATION *continued*

compressions and mouth-to-mouth ventilation.

● For a child, place the heel of one hand two finger widths above where the ribs meet on the breastbone, and press down sharply five times (see illustrations between pages 96 and 97). For a baby under 12 months, place the tips of two fingers on the lower breastbone, just below the nipple line (see illustrations between pages 96 and 97).

● Give one full breath of mouth-to-mouth ventilation.

● Continue at a rate of five chest compressions to one breath for one minute.

● Call for an ambulance.

● Continue giving CPR (five chest compressions followed by one breath of mouth-to-mouth ventilation) until the ambulance arrives.

ANIMAL BITES

DEEP OR LARGE BITE
If the wound is bleeding, apply direct pressure (use a clean handkerchief or dressing for this), holding the wound above the level of your child's heart. Cover it with a sterile dressing, if possible. Bandage firmly and take your child to hospital.

SUPERFICIAL BITE
Clean the wound thoroughly, using soap and warm water. Pat dry and cover with a dressing. Do not apply antiseptic cream.

● If your child has had all his usual injections, then he will not need a tetanus booster, but if he is bitten outside the UK seek medical help immediately, because of the risk of rabies. Remember that human bites can be just as dangerous as animal bites.

First Aid

ASTHMA ATTACK

Your child will have difficulty speaking and breathing, will wheeze on breathing out and be suffering from stress and anxiety. She may also have a grey-blue tinge to her face and lips. For a first attack you should call the doctor, or an ambulance if the attack is severe. Make sure the room is well ventilated and sit the child forward with her arms resting on a table to ease her breathing. Try to remain calm – reassure your child and do your best to help her relax.

If your child has medication for her asthma, use this as early on in the attack as you can. If the attack does not ease, call an ambulance.

BLEEDING

Apply firm pressure to the wound with, ideally, a pad (made from a dressing or handkerchief) for at least five minutes. Be as firm as possible, but ease up if you are restricting circulation (signs of this are numbness, whiteness, or pins and needles in the limb).

Keep checking the circulation beyond the bandage and, if necessary, loosen it a little. Elevate the injured part above the level of the heart if you can. But do not move or elevate the part if you suspect a fracture. For large cuts, lie the child down.

- If something like a piece of glass is embedded in the wound, don't try to remove it. Apply firm pressure on the two sides of the object and put padding around it before applying a bandage.

- If blood starts to soak through the dressing, do not take it off. Simply apply another firm dressing on top.

- Never use a tourniquet.

- Heavy bleeding (either internal or external) can cause shock; so remember your ABC of resuscitation (see page 93).

- Seek medical advice. For a very severe cut, call 999.

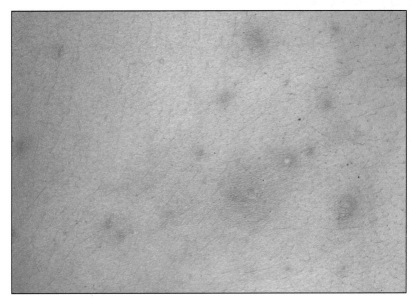

The chief symptom of **chickenpox** is a spreading, itchy rash of raised red spots, which turn to blisters before bursting and crusting over to form scabs. (*St John's Institute of Dermatology*)

Fifth disease is sometimes known as 'slapped cheek disease' because it begins with a bright red rash on the cheeks, as if they have been slapped. A fine, lacy rash then appears on the limbs and trunk. (*Collections/Kim Naylor*)

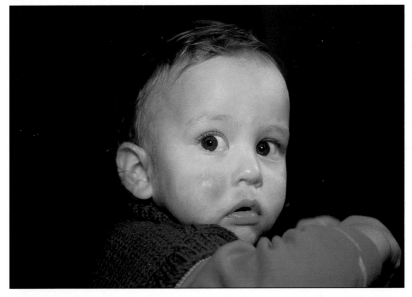

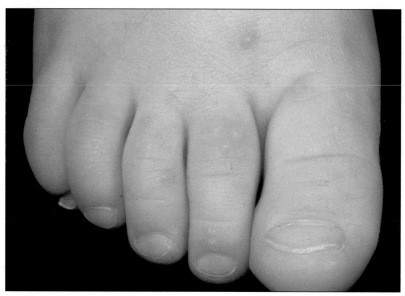

Hand, foot and mouth disease causes tiny, round blisters on the hands and feet, and sores inside the mouth, which last for a few days. (*St John's Institute of Dermatology*)

Impetigo is a highly infectious skin condition caused by bacteria getting into cracked or broken skin. The symptomatic red spots – typically starting on the face – gradually turn into fluid-filled blisters, which then crust over, and new spots form. (*St John's Institute of Dermatology*)

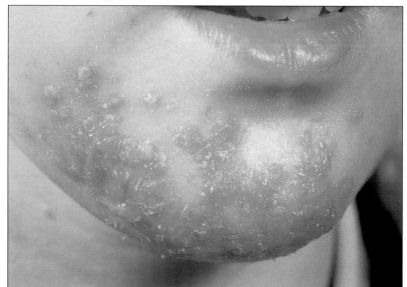

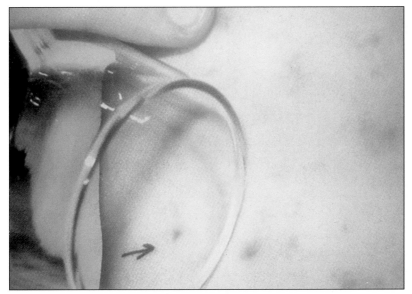

The glass tumbler test. If your child has a purple, bruise-like rash that doesn't fade when you press a drinking glass against it, it could be **meningitis**. (*Meningitis Research Foundation*)

The **rubella** rash is a pinky-red rash which starts on the face and spreads first to the trunk, then to the arms and legs. (*St John's Institute of Dermatology*)

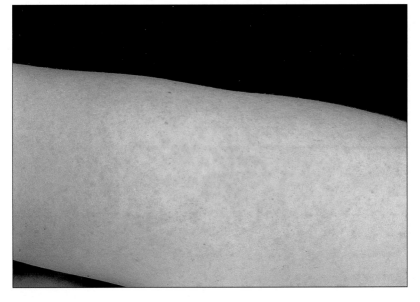

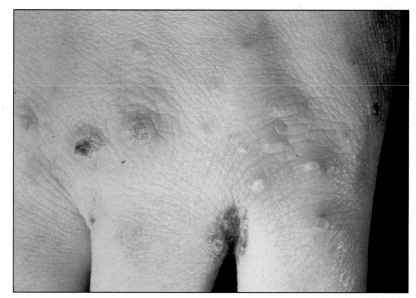

The **scabies** rash is very infectious and intensely itchy – especially at night. It is caused by an allergy to a mite that burrows under the skin, particularly the webs of skin between the fingers and the toes. (*St John's Institute of Dermatology*)

Urticaria is a very itchy raised skin rash that is almost always caused by an allergic reaction. (*Dr P. Marazzi/Science Photo Library*)

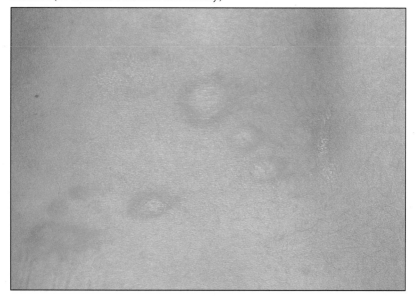

BURNS AND SCALDS

Cool the burn by pouring cold water over it for at least 10 minutes – using a shower-head in the bath is a good method of doing this, but don't immerse your child in water. And never try to remove any clothing that might be sticking to the burned area. Once the burn is cooled, simply cut around any material that might be sticking to the skin. Carefully loosen or remove any tight clothing, watches or jewellery from the area of the burn, in case it begins to swell. Don't apply lotions, fat or ointment to the burn. Just cover it with a clean plastic bag, clingfilm or a clean, non-fluffy dressing to protect it from infection and seek medical advice.

There are three types of burn:

SUPERFICIAL
Here the surface of the skin is burnt. These burns cause redness, pain and some swelling. They simply need to be kept clean and dry, and they usually don't scar.

PARTIAL THICKNESS
Deeper layers of the skin are burnt. These blister and can easily become infected as a result of this. Never attempt to burst any blisters.

FULL THICKNESS
All the layers of the skin are affected. These burns are painless, as the nerves are actually damaged. The burn looks grey and waxy, or even charred.

Call 999 for all serious burns and see a doctor for:

- All full-thickness burns

- Partial-thickness burns where the blister covers an area larger than a 50p piece

- Superficial burns that affect more than 9 per cent of the body surface. As a simple guide to working this out: the size of the palm of the child's hand equals one per cent. The whole of an arm is nine per cent, the whole of a leg or the whole of the front or back of the torso is 18 per cent. (If in doubt, seek medical help anyway)

- All burns which are on the child's face, or over any joints

- All burns to the child's mouth and throat

First Aid

CHOKING

Choking can happen when something solid – such as a lump of food – gets lodged in the trachea, which is the main airway leading into the lungs. If the object blocks off the air supply, then the body will very rapidly become starved of oxygen, and the child will suffer brain damage or die.

Signs of choking

IN A BABY

Initially her face will look flushed and then turn blue, and she'll breathe noisily or stop breathing.

IN AN OLDER CHILD

She will turn blue or very pale, have difficulty speaking, breathe noisily, or stop breathing and clutch at her throat in distress. At any age unconsciousness will follow within a few minutes.

What to do

FOR A BABY
Back slaps

Lay your baby face down along your forearm. Then with your other hand, slap her on the back between her shoulder blades (see illustrations between pages 96 and 97). (Keep your baby's head down low and support her chin.) Do this five times. If this doesn't shift the blockage, lay her face up along your other arm. Check in her mouth and take out any obstruction. If back slaps have failed, keep your baby face up along your arm and try:

Chest thrusts

Put two fingertips on the baby's breastbone (see illustrations between pages 96 and 97), about 1cm below the nipple line. Give five sharp chest compressions with your fingers. These act as artificial coughs.

Check gently in your baby's mouth to see whether the obstruction has cleared. If it hasn't, call an ambulance and keep on repeating the sequence of five slaps on the back, five chest thrusts, then checking the mouth until help arrives or the obstruction shifts.

FOR AN OLDER CHILD

Encourage your child to cough the obstruction up, but don't waste time. The next step is to try:

Back slaps

Bend a small child over your lap, or keep a larger child standing up, but make him bend well forward. Using the heel of your hand give five hard slaps to

CHOKING *continued*

the back (see illustrations), between your child's shoulder blades. If this fails, move on to:

Chest thrusts
Stand or kneel behind the child. Make a fist and place it at the lower end of the breastbone (see illustrations), and pull sharply upwards five times, at a rate of about one every three seconds. If the blockage still hasn't cleared, start:

Abdominal thrusts
These are similar to chest thrusts, but your fist pulls up into the upper central abdomen, just below the breastbone (see illustrations). Call an ambulance and keep repeating the sequence of five claps on the back, five chest thrusts, and five abdominal thrusts until help arrives or the obstruction shifts. Never use abdominal thrusts on a baby under 12 months. Keep checking whether the obstruction has shifted by gently feeling in the mouth.

If the child becomes unconscious, her throat may relax, and she may be able to breathe. Check her airway, breathing and circulation (see ABC of resuscitation, page 93). If she isn't breathing, begin resuscitation until help arrives.

CONVULSIONS

The most common causes of convulsions are fever, caused by infections, such as throat or ear infections (these are remarkably common in children under five), epilepsy, head injuries and poisoning. But sometimes convulsions occur for no apparent reason. All children who have a first convulsion should be assessed in hospital to exclude any serious cause, but for second and subsequent convulsions most children can be treated at home.

What to do

● Try to make sure that the child can't injure herself in any way by knocking against hard surfaces or objects. Put

First Aid

CONVULSIONS *continued*

pillows or cushions around her to absorb violent movements and turn her on to her side so there's no danger of inhaling any vomit.

- Loosen any tight-fitting clothing.

- There may be prolonged or repeated convulsions. When the convulsion is over, she may be unconscious, so check that her airway is open and also check for breathing and a pulse (see the ABC of resuscitation, page 93). It's common for breathing to stop for a few seconds, so try not to be alarmed, but immediately follow the ABC routine.

- If your child is breathing, place her in the recovery position and then call a doctor.

For febrile convulsions (where the child has a high fever): cool her down by removing any bedclothes, and as much clothing as is easy to get at – but don't make her too cold. Use a fan, or sponge her down with lukewarm water. Roll her on to her side and then call a doctor.

DROWNING

Get the child out of the water – carry her with her head lower than her chest to reduce the risk of inhaling water. Lie her down on something warm, remove any wet clothes and cover her with a blanket or dry clothes. If she's unconscious, you will need to assess her condition and follow the ABC of resuscitation (see page 93) – open the airway, then check for breathing and a pulse. If necessary, carry out CPR for one minute (but don't try to use abdominal thrusts), call an ambulance and continue until help arrives. If the child is breathing, place her in the recovery position until help comes.

- Don't push on the stomach to force up water that may have been swallowed. This increases the risk that it will be inhaled.

- If your child regains consciousness, keep her warm.

- Don't give up resuscitation until professional help

DROWNING *continued*

arrives. People have completely recovered after 30 minutes of appearing not to breathe (the cold slows the body down).

- Even if your child appears to recover, ensure she has a thorough medical check at the nearest hospital accident and emergency department.

ELECTRIC SHOCK

Electric shock may cause breathing – and sometimes the heart – to stop. The current may also cause burns.

FOR DOMESTIC ELECTRICITY SUPPLIES

- Don't touch the child's skin if he is still in contact with the current.

- Disconnect the electric current at the mains, or failing that, the socket. If you can't disconnect the power, stand on something that doesn't conduct electricity (such as a phone directory) and push the wire or electrical appliance away using a wooden object, like a chair or broom (see illustrations between pages 96 and 97). Alternatively, drag him away with a loop of rope around a foot, but don't touch his skin.

- Carry out the ABC of resuscitation (see page 93) and call 999.

- Treat electrical burns as you would burns from heat. Don't pour water on them unless you're sure power is off.

FOR OVERHEAD ELECTRICITY SUPPLIES

Don't try to deal with shocks from overhead powerlines. High voltage electricity can jump up to 20 yards, killing anyone who goes near. Call 999 and make sure you keep others away.

First Aid

FRACTURES

The signs of a fracture are pain, tenderness, and sometimes a grating sensation when moving, swelling or bruising around the fracture site, and loss of function, because movement is too painful or the joint is unstable.

- If you suspect your child has a fracture, try to avoid moving him, if possible. Steady and support the injured limb using cushions or folded clothes – both above and below the fracture site – or simply by holding the limb gently and keeping it still.

- Don't give your child any food or drink until the fracture has been assessed by a doctor.

- If the child is unconscious, place in the recovery position and remember the ABC of resuscitation (page 93).

- If there's a wound over the fracture, cover it with a sterile dressing, clean cloth or handkerchief, but if medical help or an ambulance is on its way, then don't try to bandage the affected part.

HEAD INJURIES

If there's a cut, you must deal with any bleeding (use firm pressure and cover it), and treat any minor bruise or bump with a cold compress such as a cloth wrung out in cold water. Also look out for signs of nausea, dizziness, complaints of changes in vision, or slight drowsiness. If any of these occur, see a doctor immediately.

Major injuries

If the child is unconscious, put her in the recovery position (see page 93). A short spell of unconsciousness is common. But even if the child recovers quickly, you must seek medical help.

- If unconsciousness lasts more than three minutes, call 999 right away, and if it persists, be prepared to do CPR (see page 94).

- If you notice a discharge from the ear, cover with a sterile or clean pad, and lie the child with that ear lower than the other.

NECK AND BACK INJURIES

- Clues that the spine is damaged include pain in the back or neck, tenderness of the spine, difficulty moving limbs, loss of sensation to part of the body, difficulty breathing, or obvious deformity of the spine.

- Do not move the child unless he is in danger (such as from fire or fumes). Try to calm him, and tell him to keep still.

- Keep the neck and spine in a straight line by holding the child's head – put your hands over the child's ears, and hold gently but firmly (see illustrations between pages 96 and 97).

- Get a helper to put padding around his neck and shoulders.

- Get someone to call 999.

- If the child is unconscious, keep his head and neck straight while turning into the recovery position. If you have to do CPR (see page 94), lift the chin without tilting the head.

POISONING

If your child has swallowed anything potentially poisonous – medication, household chemicals, berries, etc – act promptly. **Do not attempt to make your child vomit** unless instructed to do so by a doctor or paramedic. Some chemicals can do as much, or more, damage on their way up as they did on their way down.

Call 999 or your doctor immediately and give as much information as you can about the poison.

- Wipe away any residual chemical from around his mouth and if the child complains of burning lips, give sips of cold water or milk.

- If you know your child drank a corrosive poison, and he is still conscious, give water or milk to drink to dilute it in case he vomits.

- Be prepared to perform resuscitation – check your ABC of resuscitation (see

First Aid

POISONING *continued*

page 93) – if the child becomes unconscious. For corrosive poisons, give mouth-to-nose – rather than mouth-to-mouth – ventilation.

- Take any bottles, berries, plant labels or any other evidence of what the child has ingested, with you to the hospital or doctor's surgery.

ROAD ACCIDENTS

Road accidents can range from a motorway pile-up to a child falling off her bike, but a few general rules apply:

- For all serious accidents, call 999 right away.

- Think before you act – that includes making sure you're safe. Getting injured by rushing in front of a car to get to your child doesn't help anyone.

- If you're in a car when the accident happens, turn off the engine and make sure that no one is smoking.

- Don't try to move an unconscious casualty unless it's absolutely essential, and assume the neck is injured.

- Don't remove a child's helmet if she's unconscious, unless you think her airway may be blocked.

- See the advice given for head injuries, fractures or cuts and remember your ABC of resuscitation (page 93).

SHOCK

Shock results in lowered blood pressure, and its most likely cause is serious bleeding (internal or external), or severe burns or scalds, which must be treated without delay. Early signs that someone is suffering from shock are rapid pulse, sweating, cold and clammy skin, and grey-blue lips. Later the child may feel weak and giddy, thirsty and his breathing may be rapid and shallow, and his

SHOCK *continued*

pulse weak. Eventually the child may be gasping for air, become unconscious, and sometimes suffer cardiac arrest.

What to do

Lay the child down and loosen his clothing. Turn his head to one side and then raise his legs as high as possible – use several pillows or cushions to support his legs.

- Call 999 and be ready to follow the ABC of resuscitation (see page 93).

- Put a blanket or some clothing over your child if he's cold but don't apply a hot water bottle.

- Keep reassuring your child, and encourage him to talk until an ambulance arrives.

SMOKE INHALATION

A smoke-filled room can be dangerous for two main reasons. Smoke may contain poisonous gases (from burning plastics or synthetic wallcoverings, for example) which can severely irritate the lungs and even kill. Fire sucks the oxygen out of the air and leads to suffocation.

- Call 999. All victims of smoke inhalation should be checked at hospital.

- Never enter a smoke-filled room. Your life will be at risk.

- Get everyone well away from the smoky area as quickly as

you can and keep a close eye on anyone who has been exposed to smoke or fumes. They may look all right initially, but if the lining of the airways has been inflamed they may begin to choke or wheeze.

- Extinguish any clothing that is alight by wrapping the child in something non-flammable or rolling her on the ground. Remove clothing, cutting it away, if necessary.

- If the child is unconscious, follow the ABC of resuscitation (see page 93). If she's breathing, put her in the recovery position.

Flat Feet

See also Knock-Knees

An apparent absence of the normal arch on the inside of the feet. Doctors used to worry a great deal about flat feet, until someone noticed that three of the first four people to run a four-minute mile had apparently all had flat feet!

SYMPTOMS

Flat feet by themselves do not matter. They should only be a cause for concern if they cause any pain on walking. Many small children appear to have flat feet when they go through the normal stage of having knock-knees. This causes the feet to roll inwards, flattening the arch. After the age of about five years, the normal arch of the foot usually becomes visible again.

ACTION

If your child still appears to have flat feet after the age of five, ask him or her to stand on tiptoe. Usually, when a child does this the normal arch of the foot appears. If no arch appears, then further assessment may be necessary. In addition, any form of flat foot that is painful should be assessed by your GP.

USUAL TREATMENT

If a child stands on tiptoe and the arch of the foot appears, then there is no underlying problem, and the only difficulty this type of flat foot can cause is uneven wearing of the shoes. Insoles or wedges can help, but talk to your doctor about this first. He or she may make a referral to a physiotherapist or chiropodist.

Foreign Bodies

See also Cough ● Vaginal Discharge

Children have a delightful tendency to experiment, and this can sometimes lead to things getting where they shouldn't be. A foreign body may be inserted either deliberately or accidentally.

SYMPTOMS

INHALED OBJECTS
Often the child who has inhaled something will have no recollection of this. However, in any child who has been coughing for more than a couple of weeks without any other explanation (such as asthma) your doctor will consider the possibility of an inhaled foreign body blocking one of the bronchi (air tubes) and leading to irritation, inflammation and even the possible collapse of part of the lung.

OBJECTS IN THE NOSE
Nasal congestion and catarrh normally affect both sides of the nose equally. If there is a green or yellow discharge from just one side of the nose, this means that there is something irritating just that side. Your child could have stuck a small object up the nose which has caused blockage, irritation and infection.

OBJECTS IN THE EAR
A foreign body in the ear will cause pain and discharge if it becomes lodged.

OBJECTS IN THE EYE
Anything that gets into your child's eye will be immediately painful and irritating.

ACTION

INHALED OBJECTS
If you know that your child has inhaled something, and hasn't immediately coughed it up, then consult a doctor. If he or she is breathless, see First Aid (page 93), immediately and call an ambulance if the situation worsens.

For an unexplained persistent

Foreign Bodies

cough, consult your doctor. If a cough started soon after an episode of choking, even if you think the child managed to cough up whatever caused the choking, tell your doctor.

OBJECTS IN THE NOSE
If your child has just inserted something into the nose, and you know it is still there, then try to get him or her to blow the nose, if the child is old enough. If the object won't shift, *never* attempt to get it out yourself. Always see a doctor without delay.

OBJECTS IN THE EAR
Do not attempt to remove the object, even if you can see it, as you may push it further in. Consult your doctor.

OBJECTS IN THE EYE
A foreign body in the eye needs immediate treatment. Don't let your child rub the eye as this could make the situation worse. Instead, try to flush out the object using plenty of cold water. If this doesn't work, see a doctor at once.

USUAL TREATMENT

INHALED OBJECTS
The doctor will arrange a chest x-ray.

OBJECTS IN THE NOSE
Most doctors will refer your child to the Accident and Emergency department, unless they have the equipment to remove the foreign body without risking pushing it further inside.

OBJECTS IN THE EAR
The doctor may remove the object with fine tweezers or else float it out by gently syringing the ear with liquid.

OBJECTS IN THE EYE
If you have been able to wash the object out but your child's eye is red and/or painful or he or she is complaining about unusual vision, you should go to the Accident and Emergency department.

Foreskin Problems

See also Hypospadias

All boys are born with a foreskin that covers the glans, or tip, of the penis. Many problems result from parents who forcefully pull back the foreskin to clean under it. This risks scarring which will cause problems later. The most common foreskin problem is that it is too tight, restricting the normal urine flow.

SYMPTOMS

In some boys the foreskin does not retract completely until the age of 10 years. If it has been pulled back forcefully, it can become stuck behind the head of the penis, where it swells up. This condition is known as paraphimosis. As the foreskin swells, it squeezes on the penis, which also swells, and eventually the normal flow of urine is restricted. If the foreskin is too tight, urine sprays all over the place and the foreskin balloons out. Sometimes the foreskin will swell up in its normal position. This can be caused if it is trapped in a zip, or by poor hygiene or by soap being left under the foreskin after washing.

ACTION

If the foreskin is swollen, tender and has pus oozing out, or there are signs of paraphimosis, then seek medical help. If it is swollen but painless and not particularly red, gentle soaking with warm water can help. Do *not* add bubble bath or use soap.

USUAL TREATMENT

Inflammation of the glans of the penis may need antibiotics, and a persistently tight foreskin may indicate the need for circumcision.

Fractures

A fracture is a crack or break in a bone. As children's bones are still growing, a relatively minor crack can affect the way the bone grows, so should be taken seriously. The most common fractures in young children are called greenstick fractures. Rather than the bone cracking right through, it splits like a piece of green twig when you try and snap it.

SYMPTOMS

The signs of a fracture are pain, tenderness, and sometimes a grating sensation on movement, swelling or bruising around the fracture site, and loss of function, because the child finds movement is too painful or the joint is unstable.

ACTION

If the fracture has just happened, emergency treatment is needed. See First Aid, page 102, for what to do.

USUAL TREATMENT

Possible fractures will always need assessing by a doctor, ideally at an Accident and Emergency unit. An x-ray will confirm whether there is a fracture. Not all fractures require a plaster cast but many do in order to immobilize the broken limb. After the cast has been fitted, your child can usually go home and you will be given advice on painkillers. There will probably be a follow-up appointment at the hospital fracture clinic within the next few days to check that the cast is comfortable and that the injury is healing. If your child is in discomfort or his or her toes or fingers have swollen or become darker, the cast may be too tight and you should mention this to the team at the clinic. Serious fractures may require surgery to rejoin the bones.

Fungal Infections

See also Nappy Rash ● Ringworm ● Scalp Problems

Fungi have nothing to do with mushrooms! Fungi can affect almost any area of the skin, in particular parts not exposed to the air. They cause conditions such as ringworm, seborrhoeic dermatitis of the scalp and athlete's foot. The first two of these conditions are dealt with elsewhere, but athlete's foot has many of the typical symptoms of a fungal infection. Thrush is another common fungal infection which most often affects the mouth or nappy area of young children.

SYMPTOMS

ATHLETE'S FOOT
This infection usually occurs when fungi get between the toes where the skin may become cracked and soggy. Usually the webs between the fourth and fifth toes are affected. This can cause an annoying itch so that the child then scratches the area, which then worsens the condition. Sometimes blisters occur. The sole and instep areas can also be affected.

THRUSH
Thrush is caused by a fungus known as *Candida albicans* which thrives anywhere in the body that is warm and moist. Thrush in the mouth produces white patches inside the cheeks and on the tongue. These can occasionally be quite sore and may interfere with the baby's feeding. They look like dried patches of milk, but unlike milk they cannot be wiped away.

ACTION

ATHLETE'S FOOT
Like all similar fungal infections, the fungus that causes athlete's foot thrives on warm, damp conditions. The first step in clearing the infection is to keep the skin dry and well ventilated. Many children wear trainers that

Fungal Infections

don't allow the skin to breathe, particularly in warm weather, and which are a perfect environment for the development of this condition. Leaving the feet exposed to the air helps a great deal. If the weather is warm, sandals without socks are ideal footwear as they let the air circulate. Athlete's foot is contagious, so you should make sure your child uses separate towels and flannels from the rest of the family.

Fungal infections on the skin in other places apart from on the feet can be difficult to diagnose. If you are not sure whether your child has a fungal infection or eczema, then consult your doctor before attempting to treat the problem. If you use anti-eczema creams on a fungal infection, for instance, you may make the condition worse so it is always a good idea to get a correct diagnosis.

THRUSH
If you suspect that your child has got thrush, contact your doctor or health visitor for treatment. This is certainly not an emergency, and children frequently have no symptoms at all.

USUAL TREATMENT

ATHLETE'S FOOT
Make sure that your child's feet are thoroughly washed and then completely dried, especially between the toes. Apply anti-fungal creams twice a day. Never use any form of steroid cream to treat athlete's foot without your doctor's advice.

THRUSH
Thrush is usually treated with an anti-fungal suspension, such as nystatin, or a gel, such as Daktarin. These are usually applied about four times a day until the lesions have cleared up. Even if you are a sufferer from vaginal thrush, it is most unlikely that you will have passed this infection on to your child.

Gastroenteritis

See also Dehydration ● Diarrhoea ● Vomiting

An inflammation of the bowel, causing diarrhoea and/or vomiting. Most gastroenteritis infections are caused by viruses, particularly a virus known as rotavirus. However, they are sometimes caused by bacteria and other organisms, as in the case of food poisoning. The only way to tell whether an infection is caused by a virus or bacteria is by laboratory examination of a stool specimen.

SYMPTOMS

The main symptom is diarrhoea, often watery, and often accompanied by vomiting, and sometimes a raised temperature and abdominal pain. Dehydration can be a problem.

ACTION

Contact your doctor urgently if you think your child is dehydrated, which is much more likely if the child is also vomiting. You should also always contact a doctor if your child has bloody diarrhoea. If symptoms continue for more than 24 hours without showing any sign of improving, then at least contact your doctor for advice.

USUAL TREATMENT

Prevent dehydration by giving fluids. Children with profuse diarrhoea who are reluctant to drink should be given special rehydration powders and avoid milk. Antibiotics will usually have no effect and may make the diarrhoea worse.

Growing Pains

See also Arthritis ● Limping

Pains in the limbs, particularly the legs, affect about 10 per cent of children aged between four and eight years old. Growth in itself doesn't hurt, so the name is rather misleading.

SYMPTOMS

No one fully understands these pains, which are often felt deep in the thigh or lower leg. They are fairly uncommon during the day, causing most pain in the evening and night and they can be bad enough to wake your child at night. Even though they can be quite severe, and even bad enough to make a child cry with discomfort, they are not associated with any detectable underlying abnormality, or with limping or swelling of the joints.

ACTION

If your child complains of pains in just one leg, rather than both, or if the pain causes limping or fever, or if there are specific tender areas on the legs, then consult your doctor. You should also consult your doctor if your child complains that the pain is always coming from a joint, rather than the muscles. These are unlikely to be simple growing pains, and it is important that your doctor assesses your child and rules out any other cause.

USUAL TREATMENT

Reassurance, a warm hot water bottle and gently rubbing the legs will help. Occasionally paracetamol may help. Growing pains themselves never lead to any long-term damage to the bones or muscles.

Growth Disorders

Growth can be affected by many factors, such as hormones, diet or illness. It is important to consult your doctor if you think that growth does not seem to be continuing at the right pace.

WHAT TO WATCH FOR

Monitoring your child's rate of growth is extremely important. While children obviously vary greatly in their individual sizes, it should be possible to predict and monitor how well they are growing. This is done using centile charts. Imagine standing your child in a row of 100 children of the same sex who were born on the day that your child was born. Imagine them lined up from the smallest at one end to the tallest at the other. If your child is forty-fifth along the line today, he or she should still be about forty-fifth in a few months' time. If growth is poor, then the position in the line (known as the centile) will have changed, and this should alert the doctor or health visitor to assess possible causes.

ACTION

Consult your doctor or health visitor if you think your child isn't growing as he should be.

USUAL TREATMENT

Growth can be affected by poorly controlled long-term illnesses such as asthma, or by problems affecting absorption of nutrients, such as coeliac disease. Sometimes the problem is a shortage of growth hormone. A thorough medical assessment will be required, together with on-going monitoring.

Hair Loss

See also Scalp Problems

Children sometimes develop one or more patches of baldness, a condition known as alopecia areata. The cause is unknown.

SYMPTOMS

Hair loss in small patches can occur on a scalp that is otherwise completely healthy. These patches are often oval in shape and are not associated with any itching or other inflammation of the scalp. They are usually discovered by parents, but it is extremely unusual for hair loss to spread.

Patches of hair loss are not of any important medical significance, provided your child is otherwise fit and well. General thinning of the hair, as opposed to patches of hair loss, can occasionally suggest a lack of thyroid hormone, usually accompanied by lethargy and obesity.

ACTION

If the bald patches are small and easily covered by other hair, don't worry about them, and don't bother with any treatments or lotions. If the patches are getting larger, or the scalp is itchy or inflamed, then consult your doctor. Irritating scalp conditions such as eczema may make your child scratch his or her scalp and this could result in loss of hair.

USUAL TREATMENT

Most alopecia areata needs no treatment at all. The hair almost always begins to regrow spontaneously in time. Do not be tempted to purchase lotions that are designed to stimulate hair growth. Most of these are useless and should not be used on children.

Hand, Foot and Mouth Disease

A viral infection causing blisters on the hands and feet, and sores in the mouth. It has no connection with the cattle disease.

SYMPTOMS

The illness may start with a slight temperature, sore throat, or abdominal pains, followed by a rash of tiny round blisters (see pages 160–2 and illustration between pages 128 and 129) which usually affects the palms of the hands, the tips of the fingers, the inside of the mouth, and the soles and outside edges of the feet. The rash lasts for a few days and then fades away.

ACTION

Unless you are certain of the diagnosis, then go to see your doctor. Sores in the mouth in babies might be mistaken for thrush, so it is a good idea to double-check.

USUAL TREATMENT

No particular treatment is required. The sore mouth can make eating and drinking very uncomfortable so, if this is the case, use paracetamol. If your child cannot swallow this, ask your doctor or pharmacist about suppositories. Some older children are able to use a mouthwash, though don't give this if there is a risk that your child may swallow it. The incubation period of hand, foot and mouth disease is between three and five days. Children with this condition are infectious during the period of the illness, and should be kept off school until they are well.

Hayfever

See also Allergies ● Conjunctivitis

Hayfever rarely has anything to do with hay, and certainly doesn't cause a fever. It is also known as seasonal rhinitis. Rhinitis means inflammation of the nose. Many children have hayfever-type symptoms year round, and this is then known as perennial (year-round) rhinitis.

SEASONAL RHINITIS
This frequently runs in families, and is caused by an allergy to certain grasses, trees or weeds. These plants depend on the wind for cross-pollination and release their pollen into the air. Pollen allergies usually occur in the spring or early summer. The months in which your child experiences symptoms depends on which type of pollen causes the allergy, as different plants produce pollen at different times of the year. Symptoms are likely to be worst in dry, windy weather when more pollens and spores are in the air.

PERENNIAL RHINITIS
This condition can be triggered off by an allergy to almost anything that is present year round, but the most common triggers are house dust or house-dust mites, animals, birds, moulds, chemicals or plants. Sometimes no obvious cause can be found. If your doctor diagnoses a house-dust mite allergy, this does not mean that you do not keep your house clean. You only have to look at a shaft of sunlight streaming through a window to realize how many dust particles there are – even in the cleanest house. House-dust mites live on dust, and are extremely common.

Hayfever

SYMPTOMS

The chief symptoms are sneezing, a constantly runny or congested nose, an itchy nose, and often watering and itchy eyes.

ACTION

Hayfever is not an emergency, but talk to your doctor, who will make a full assessment of possible causes, may be able to provide information sheets, and can prescribe treatment. Skin tests may determine the exact cause for the allergy, but this is certainly not always essential or indeed particularly helpful. Discovering the exact cause of the allergy can be helpful if it allows your child to avoid the trigger substance, but there is little to be gained from pinpointing the exact pollen, for instance, if your child cannot avoid exposure to it. It does mean, however, that you might be able to identify when an allergy might be at its worst and take precautions in advance.

USUAL TREATMENT

SEASONAL RHINITIS
Try to make sure that – as far as possible – your child avoids contact with whatever he or she is allergic to. For example, if you know that the allergy is brought on by fresh flowers during the pollen season, then don't bring fresh flowers into the house. However, if tree pollens are the cause of your child's symptoms, then avoidance is near impossible.

PERENNIAL RHINITIS
For children with perennial rhinitis, house-dust mite is the most frequent culprit. To control this, try any or all of the following measures:

● Get rid of any old or musty furniture that may be harbouring dust, mould, or dust mites.

Hayfever

USUAL TREATMENT *continued*

- Vacuum soft furnishings, carpets, rugs and mattresses frequently.

- Consider fitting special mattress and pillow covers that are designed specifically to help keep dust down.

- In the bedroom, use foam rather than feather pillows, damp-dust the room every two or three days, and try to avoid clutter in the room.

- Consider banning pets from the main living areas. If your child turns out to be allergic to a pet, then you have a very difficult decision to make – but don't forget that the trauma of losing the pet may be worse than the drawbacks of the allergy.

- Avoid toys that might collect dust and cannot be washed.

Finally, make your house a no-smoking zone. There is no doubt at all that smoke worsens the symptoms of rhinitis in all sufferers.

Inflammation in the nose can be reduced very successfully using nasal sprays such as Beconase, Flixonase or Syntaris that contain a very small dose of steroid. They have to be used on a regular daily basis, but can be extremely effective. The dosage of steroid involved is extremely small to cause any significant side-effects. Don't stop using them the moment your child seems better but ask your doctor's advice on how long to keep using them. An alternative, non-steroid treatment contains disodium cromoglycate, a chemical that can block histamine release. It has to be used far more frequently than the steroid sprays and is usually not quite as effective.

Antihistamines are the most commonly used treatments. Their great advantage is that they usually deal with all aspects of the allergy throughout the body. So, if your child has eye symptoms as well as nose symptoms, the same medication will frequently deal with both conditions. The older antihistamines tended to have a rather sedative effect, but newer drugs have far fewer side-effects. Many children start with one approach, such as an antihistamine, and only add or substitute other therapies if this does not seem to be working well enough.

There is no cure for hayfever, although most children will eventually grow out of it.

Head-Banging

See also Terrible Twos

Surprisingly, many children, especially toddlers, are head-bangers, and repeatedly bang their head against the floor or bed.

WHAT TO WATCH FOR

Head-banging always looks very dramatic and sometimes frightening, and is often very worrying for parents who are concerned that it must be the sign of some major emotional disturbance. After all, if you or I were to bang our heads in the same way that many small children do, we would probably have a terrible headache, a bruised forehead and a liking for heavy metal music. However, children are quite different. They seem to enjoy it and almost never damage themselves.

ACTION

This is a problem that always bothers parents more than children. The best approach is to try and work out why he or she is doing it. Parents often find that there is some sort of trigger, such as boredom or frustration, and if you can deal with this, then your child will be very likely to abandon the habit soon enough. However, some children just do it for no obvious reason.

USUAL TREATMENT

This condition almost always gets better spontaneously in children who otherwise seem well. However, if it worries you, talk to your doctor or health visitor. In addition, if this is part of a pattern of other behavioural problems, definitely seek medical advice.

Head Lice

See also Scalp Problems

Head lice are tiny parasitic insects, approximately 3–4mm long, which only live in and on human hair. They are spread by direct contact, or by shared hats, combs or brushes.

SYMPTOMS

Usually there is itching at the back and sides of the head. It's difficult to spot the head lice unless you use a fine-toothed comb to remove them. What you may also see are their eggs, or 'nits'. Nits are white or light pink, and are usually found at the base of individual hairs.

ACTION

If you detect head lice on your child, immediately check the whole family by combing their hair, while damp, with a special fine-toothed comb which you can buy from any pharmacy. Using conditioner makes combing easier. Then treat only the person or people affected, but check the rest of the family regularly. Wash all bedding on a hot cycle. Do not treat babies under six months of age without seeking medical advice first.

USUAL TREATMENT

Ask your pharmacist about which treatment, usually a lotion, is currently being advised in your area. A local policy is often used to avoid lice developing resistance to several preparations at the same time. If the problem persists, talk to your health visitor rather than using the same lotion repeatedly. She may be able to advise you on alternative treatments.

Headache

See also Meningitis

Headaches are remarkably common in children. Estimates suggest that nearly a quarter of primary school children suffer occasional headaches, and over all ages probably one child in ten suffers from migraine. Most headaches are harmless.

SYMPTOMS

There are a number of different types of headache. Simple headaches are very common and can be caused by viral infections, fever, not drinking enough liquids or tiredness.

TENSION HEADACHES
These can be caused by almost any form of upset, tension or excitement, and are usually felt either at the front or as a band round the head. Both sides of the head tend to be affected equally and at the same time.

MIGRAINES
A migraine usually affects one side of the head. Often running in families, it may be accompanied by nausea, tummy ache or vomiting. Some children have recurrent tummy aches for months or years before the headaches start. The migraine headache itself may start with visual symptoms such as spots in front of the eyes, zig-zag lines, or even a sensation that part of the area of vision is missing. There can also be numbness or pins and needles in an arm or leg, again usually coming on before the headache.

OTHER HEADACHES
Sinusitis (inflammation of the sinuses, the passages behind the forehead and cheekbones) can cause headaches in older children, but this is not such a common problem in young children because the sinuses are less developed. **Meningitis** causes a severe pain that comes on fairly suddenly in a child who is otherwise unwell. Finally, **brain tumour** is a possible diagnosis but these are in fact extremely rare, affecting only 0.005 per cent of all children.

Headache

ACTION

If your child has a sudden, very severe headache, or a less severe headache that keeps returning or never completely goes away, see your doctor.

SUDDEN HEADACHES

Consult a doctor IMMEDIATELY if your child has any of the following:

- Headache following a head injury
- Confusion, unusual behaviour
- Vomiting more than once
- Stiff neck
- Severe pain – the child will probably scream with pain
- The pain gets worse despite paracetamol
- Headache that lasts more than 12 hours
- Reluctance to be moved
- Tries to avoid the light
- Blurred vision

RECURRENT HEADACHES

Always consult your doctor for your child's recurrent headaches if:

- The pain is usually one-sided
- Your child seems in any other way to be unwell
- The headaches are worse in the morning
- Your child is under five

USUAL TREATMENT

For most children the most useful medication for the pain of headaches is paracetamol, but it is important to give it early enough. Migraines can sometimes be prevented by dietary adjustment, by careful calculation of what the causes might be, or by the use of preventive drugs such as pizotifen (Sanomigran) or beta blockers. Reassuring your child and dealing with any anxieties and fears is also extremely important.

Heart Conditions

There is a wide variety of congenital heart conditions, frequently caused by a problem with the heart valves. The most common signs and symptoms of heart disorders are heart murmurs. Heart problems in childhood are not in any way connected with coronary artery disease, the main heart problem that affects adults.

SYMPTOMS

Symptoms of a heart disorder include abnormalities of the heart's rhythm (such as palpitations), breathlessness, or blueness of the skin and particularly the lips. However, the range of different conditions is vast. Some heart conditions cause major problems from the moment of birth, while others are completely symptom-free. About half of all babies have a soft heart murmur that can be heard using a stethoscope. When the doctor listens to the heart sounds, he or she will hear the sounds of the chambers in the heart contracting, and also the sounds of the heart valves opening and closing. Other additional sounds are known as murmurs; the great majority are entirely harmless, and are not linked with any symptoms at all. The more common harmless murmurs are caused by a whooshing of the blood as it passes from the left ventricle into the aorta, a sound which can be easily heard through a child's thin chest. Significant murmurs are usually caused by congenital heart abnormalities in which the blood can either be heard flowing through a small hole between two of the heart's chambers, or through narrowed valves.

ACTION

If you are concerned that your child has a heart problem, your doctor will first listen to the heart with a stethoscope, and then, if necessary, arrange other investigations such as a chest x-ray or ECG (echocardiogram) to pinpoint exactly what the problem is, and what needs to be done. If your doctor says your

Heart Conditions

ACTION *continued*

child has a murmur, remember that the enormous majority of these will turn out to be of no significance. Your doctor may want to investigate the murmur just to make absolutely certain that no treatment is needed.

USUAL TREATMENT

Treatment will depend to a great extent on the exact condition. Nowadays, most murmurs are checked using ultrasound or other tests which are simple and harmless. Doctors will also often keep an eye on a child until the murmur has disappeared, just to make certain that it will not be of any significance. If a murmur is thought to indicate a problem, your doctor will discuss it with you. If there is a problem with a heart valve, your child will need to be given antibiotics before any dental work is done. This is to prevent any infection from the teeth getting into the bloodstream and affecting a damaged valve.

If your child is diagnosed as having a heart condition, then find out as much information about this as you can. Ask your specialist for information.

Hernia

See also Umbilical Cord Problems

A weakness in the muscle wall of the abdomen, through which some of the contents of the abdominal cavity – usually part of the intestines – may stick out and produce a bump. While hernias in adults are usually the result of straining, in children they are usually a result of a congenital weakness.

SYMPTOMS

The most common hernias cause a swelling which comes and goes in the groin or elsewhere on the abdominal wall. Sometimes the swelling may extend into the scrotum in boys. A hernia is usually more visible when the child stands up. This is simply the effect of gravity on the abdominal contents. A hernia is only a problem if it becomes strangulated. When this happens, part of the bowel is trapped in the hernia, and this leads to blockage of the bowel (called an 'intestinal obstruction'). The main sign of strangulation is a hard swelling in the groin that won't disappear. As well as pain, there is also nausea, or vomiting.

ACTION

Consult your doctor. This is not an emergency unless the hernia is strangulated and won't go back into the abdomen.

USUAL TREATMENT

Any hernia in the groin should be repaired by surgery to prevent later strangulation occurring.

Hip Problems

See also Limping

Hip problems are quite common in childhood. A number of different conditions can cause pain or problems with the hip joints, such as **irritable hip**, an inflammation problem, or **Perthes' disease**. In Perthes' disease, the blood supply to the growing part of the upper thigh bone (the femur) becomes reduced, and the bone becomes softened and inflamed. The diseased part of the bone dies, and as the femur grows this damaged bone is replaced by new bone. The aim of treatment is to protect this newly growing bone.

Congenital dislocation of the hip (CDH) is tested for at birth. CDH affects more girls than boys, and there may well be a family history of the condition. The hip joint is a ball-and-socket joint, and if the ball and socket do not fit together correctly, the ball can slide out of the socket. Doctors test for CDH by manipulating the newborn baby's thighs to see if the joint clicks. By no means do all babies with 'clicky hips' turn out to have CDH, but it is at least a sign that more investigation is required.

SYMPTOMS

Your child may complain of pain in either the hip or the knee on the same side, limp or be reluctant to walk.

IRRITABLE HIP
A common cause of limping in small children may follow a viral infection and is caused by an inflammation of the synovium, or lining of the hip joint.

PERTHES' DISEASE
This is a less common but more serious condition. It occurs in children aged between 4 and 10 years, and usually affects only one hip. The initial symptom is of

WHAT TO DO IF A CHILD
IS UNCONSCIOUS BUT IS BREATHING AND HAS A PULSE

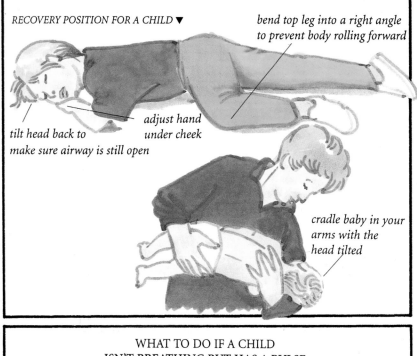

RECOVERY POSITION FOR A CHILD ▼

*bend top leg into a right angle
to prevent body rolling forward*

*adjust hand
under cheek*

*tilt head back to
make sure airway is still open*

*cradle baby in your
arms with the
head tilted*

WHAT TO DO IF A CHILD
ISN'T BREATHING BUT HAS A PULSE

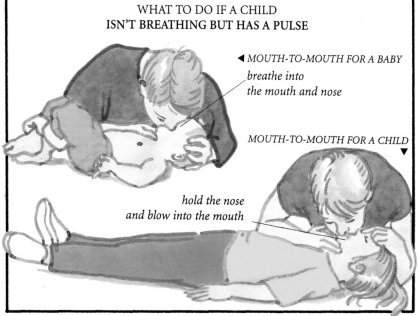

◀ *MOUTH-TO-MOUTH FOR A BABY*
*breathe into
the mouth and nose*

MOUTH-TO-MOUTH FOR A CHILD
▼

*hold the nose
and blow into the mouth*

WHAT TO DO IF A CHILD ISN'T BREATHING AND THERE IS NO PULSE

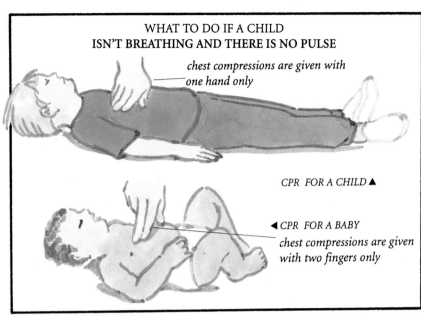

chest compressions are given with one hand only

CPR FOR A CHILD ▲

◄ *CPR FOR A BABY*
chest compressions are given with two fingers only

WHAT TO DO IF **A BABY IS CHOKING**

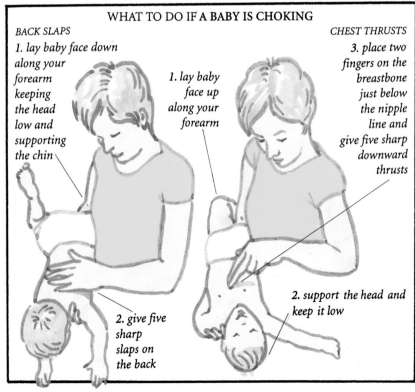

BACK SLAPS

1. lay baby face down along your forearm keeping the head low and supporting the chin

1. lay baby face up along your forearm

CHEST THRUSTS

3. place two fingers on the breastbone just below the nipple line and give five sharp downward thrusts

2. give five sharp slaps on the back

2. support the head and keep it low

WHAT TO DO IF AN OLDER CHILD IS CHOKING

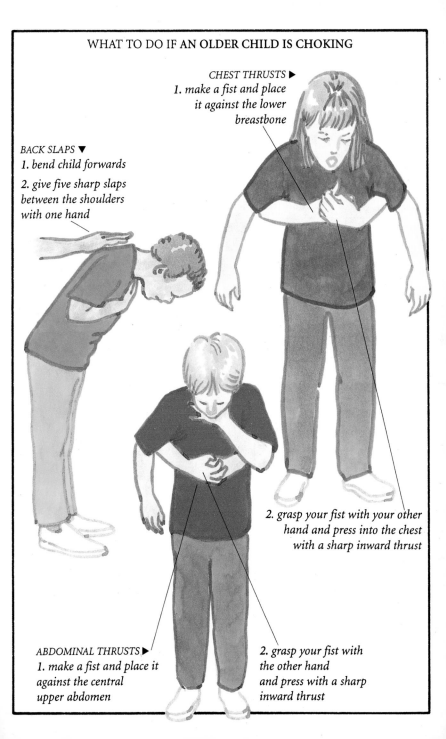

CHEST THRUSTS ▶
1. make a fist and place it against the lower breastbone

BACK SLAPS ▼
1. bend child forwards

2. give five sharp slaps between the shoulders with one hand

2. grasp your fist with your other hand and press into the chest with a sharp inward thrust

ABDOMINAL THRUSTS ▶
1. make a fist and place it against the central upper abdomen

2. grasp your fist with the other hand and press with a sharp inward thrust

WHAT TO DO IF A CHILD GETS AN ELECTRIC SHOCK

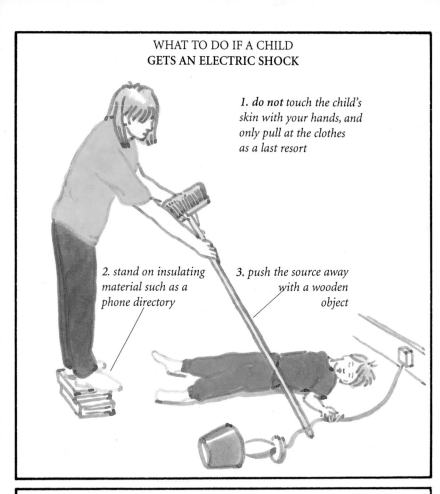

*1. **do not** touch the child's skin with your hands, and only pull at the clothes as a last resort*

2. stand on insulating material such as a phone directory

3. push the source away with a wooden object

HOW TO MOVE A CHILD WITH NECK AND BACK INJURIES

(only move if child is in danger)

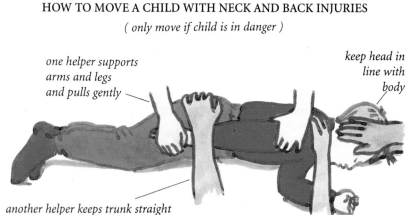

one helper supports arms and legs and pulls gently

keep head in line with body

another helper keeps trunk straight

Hip Problems

SYMPTOMS *continued*

limping; the child then complains of slight pain either in the hip or the knee.

CONGENITAL DISLOCATION OF THE HIP
If, while changing your baby's nappy, you notice a click or a clunk as you move the thighs, particularly while opening them out, then this may be a sign of a problem with the hip joint. Ask your doctor or health visitor to examine your baby.

ACTION

If your child limps for no apparent cause, or complains of pain in the hip or leg for no obvious reason, then talk to your doctor. If the pain is associated with a fever, then you should contact your doctor right away. Always seek help if the pain is severe or lasts more than a day.

USUAL TREATMENT

Irritable hip usually settles with rest but your doctor may arrange an x-ray to make sure that the hip is otherwise normal. **Perthes' disease** will need more detailed assessment, scanning, and possibly prolonged rest or, in some cases, surgery. With early treatment the outlook is excellent. In the case of **CDH**, early detection of the condition can prevent long-term problems with the hip joint and with walking. The diagnosis may be confirmed using ultrasound scanning and a full orthopaedic assessment. Treatment usually involves splinting for two to four months to hold the hip joint in its socket as it grows. This is frequently enough to lead to a total cure, with no long-lasting problems. However, in cases which are not discovered until later, traction and perhaps surgery may be required.

Hydrocephalus

An over-enlargement of the head developing around the time of birth that affects brain functioning. The brain is normally surrounded by a fluid called cerebrospinal fluid (CSF). If there is too much CSF, either due to a blockage or a failure of reabsorption, the head enlarges too rapidly.

SYMPTOMS

In babies with hydrocephalus, the fontanelle, or soft spot on the head, enlarges and may bulge, the joins between the skull bones separate, and the head becomes abnormally large. If the condition is not treated, further symptoms, such as lethargy, epilepsy and vomiting, can result from the increased pressure on the brain. Without treatment the condition can be fatal.

ACTION

Your baby's head will be measured either at or after birth, but if at any stage you are concerned about the size of your child's head, consult your doctor or health visitor. Antenatal ultrasound assessments sometimes pick up the condition before birth, and scans after birth will be able to confirm the condition.

USUAL TREATMENT

Treatment is surgical. A shunt – a tube with a valve – is inserted to allow CSF to flow from around the brain, usually to a cavity within the abdomen. Without this form of treatment there is a real risk of brain damage. If your child needs this form of operation you will be given a great deal of information about the condition and how the shunt works.

Hyperactivity

While all small children tend to be very active, some are much more active than others and these children are sometimes termed hyperactive. True hyperactivity is relatively uncommon and is associated with cases in which children have real difficulty in paying attention to what they are doing. Hyperactivity usually begins at about 18 months, and becomes more noticeable by the age of three years, with more than half the cases recognized before the age of four. It is seen more commonly in boys than girls.

SYMPTOMS

Hyperactivity is sometimes simply used as a label by parents who find their children to be uncontrollable or exceptionally boisterous. However, you should remember that almost all small children go through a phase of being constantly on the go. Describing these children as hyperactive would not be accurate – they are just being boisterous. Truly hyperactive children have a greatly reduced ability to pay attention without getting distracted. They also tend to be impulsive and overactive. The truly hyperactive child is always hyperactive, not just when he is in a certain situation. The child who appears hyperactive to his or her parents, but who behaves quite differently at playgroup, school or with grandparents is not hyperactive. This is more likely to be a behavioural problem than a medical condition.

ACTION

If you think your child may be hyperactive, talk to your GP or health visitor. It is important to try to unravel the cause. While there is no doubt that some children are genuinely hyperactive, harm may be done by labelling others erroneously. It has been suggested that certain substances in food, such as food colourings or artificial sweeteners, can cause hyperactive

Hyperactivity

behaviour. However, it is very important not to try exclusion diets, which can sometimes be of help, until the diagnosis has been confirmed. If you do try a diet and find it of no use, do not put your child on increasingly strict diets as this will do more harm than good.

Hyperactive children can be exhausting for parents, and one expert has said that the most important things we can offer children with hyperactivity are love, acceptance, respect and empathy. Some of these children are highly intelligent and are often highly creative and intuitive. However, they often do not reach their true potential, and underachieve because of their poor concentration, and the inevitable disruption of their learning. For this reason it is important to ask for expert advice from your doctor.

USUAL TREATMENT

Once the condition has been confirmed, the main treatment for overactive children is by helping parents and teachers to develop the child's concentration skills, and to increase their self-esteem. Your doctor may refer your child to a child psychologist or family therapy centre for help, which will probably consist of teaching certain patterns of behaviour. This must be tailored to the individual family's needs. In addition, stimulant medication (such as Ritalin) may be prescribed for some children with full attention-deficit hyperactivity syndrome and this can make a remarkable difference in the right cases, increasing concentration span and reducing impulsive behaviour.

Hypospadias

A congenital abnormality of the penis that affects approximately 3 in every 1000 baby boys. There are many degrees of hypospadias, but the main problem is that the urethra does not open at the tip of the glans of the penis. The urethral opening may just be a short distance from where it would normally be, or can be almost anywhere along the length of the penis towards the scrotum.

SYMPTOMS

Less serious cases of hypospadias have no symptoms at all, but with more severe forms urine will obviously flow out of the abnormal opening when your child urinates. This does not matter if the child is in nappies, but will certainly matter as he gets older. It would also have implications for sexual intercourse in years to come. In severe forms of hypospadias there may also be a problem called chordee, a marked curvature of the penis which becomes most apparent on erection.

ACTION

If you suspect that your child may have hypospadias, ask your doctor to examine him to determine whether there is a problem, and what needs to be done.

USUAL TREATMENT

Very minor problems may not need any treatment but more serious types will need surgery to reposition the urethral opening so that the boy will be able to pass urine standing up and also to ensure that erection is straight. Boys with hypospadias should not be circumcized, as the skin of the foreskin may be needed at the operation. Surgery is usually extremely successful.

Impetigo

See also Rashes

Impetigo is a highly infectious skin condition, caused by either staphylococci or streptococci bacteria.

SYMPTOMS

If skin becomes cracked or broken, bacteria can get into it, causing red spots. These gradually enlarge until they are anything up to 2cm (¾in) or more in size. They eventually turn into fluid-filled blisters. The blisters then break down, the fluid drains away, the surface crusts over, and new sore spots form (see pages 160–2, and illustration between pages 128 and 129), and the original problem gets worse. Impetigo usually starts on the face but can spread anywhere by touch. When the surface of the spot is broken, the condition is highly infectious and outbreaks can rapidly go round playgroups and schools.

ACTION

Your child should always be seen by your doctor or a nurse practitioner. This is not because impetigo is particularly serious, but because of the risk of it spreading. Make sure your child's nails are short and clean to discourage scratching.

USUAL TREATMENT

Treatment is usually with antibiotics, either as a medicine or as a cream or ointment, although some very mild cases may be treated with antiseptic creams. Make sure that each family member uses a separate flannel and towel. Children with impetigo should be kept off school for 48 hours after antibiotic treatment has been started.

Insect Bites and Stings

See also Allergy ● First Aid

A bite or sting from an insect such as a wasp, bee or mosquito usually contains a toxin, or mild poison, which can irritate the skin and occasionally produce a generalized reaction.

SYMPTOMS

Most reactions are only at the site of the bite or sting ('localized'), and cause pain, itching and swelling around the area. Occasionally children may have a severe reaction throughout the body ('generalized') or go into anaphylactic shock, with swollen itchy eyes, wheezing, nausea and abdominal pain.

ACTION

Try to remove the sting by gently scraping with your clean fingernail, or with the edge of a sterile blade. Wash the area carefully afterwards. Applying ice to the area (an ice lolly is ideal) can be soothing. Calamine lotion can help soothe particularly itchy mosquito bites. Seek advice for multiple stings, or any sting affecting the mouth. If this occurs, sucking ice may help.

For a severe generalized or anaphylactic reaction, call 999 immediately, see First Aid, page 104, and apply ice to prevent the toxin from spreading.

USUAL TREATMENT

A few children become very sensitive to bee stings and may have a severe reaction or go into anaphylactic shock when stung. Your doctor may provide a pre-loaded adrenaline syringe for emergency treatment.

Intussusception

See also Colic ● Tummy Ache

In this condition, part of the bowel telescopes inside itself. The bowel reacts by creating increasing muscular spasm, as if it were trying to move the swelling along and out, but this simply has the effect of making the problem worse.

SYMPTOMS

The symptoms of intussusception include severe colicky abdominal pain which comes in waves and causes the baby to scream, become pale, and draw his or her legs up. This is associated with vomiting and diarrhoea, swelling of the abdomen and particularly with very bloody motions (often described as 'redcurrant jelly stools'). Intussusception can follow an episode of gastro-enteritis or an upper respiratory infection which has caused enlarged glands in the abdomen.

ACTION

If your baby is aged between 3 and 12 months and appears to have severe abdominal pain and particularly if she passes bloody stools, contact your doctor immediately.

USUAL TREATMENT

Your child will need to be assessed at hospital, and an x-ray will help to confirm the diagnosis. Three-quarters of cases will be successfully treated by the bowel being pushed back into its normal position using either a special enema, or liquid, that is passed into the bowel via the anus, or by air being blown inside. The remaining quarter will need surgical treatment.

Jaundice

Most often seen in newborn babies, jaundice causes the skin and the whites of the eyes to turn a yellowish colour due to an excess of bilirubin, one of the bile pigments naturally produced as blood cells are made. In older children or adults the liver helps to remove this from the blood, but in newborn babies the liver is not fully mature, and bilirubin stays in the blood for longer.

SYMPTOMS

In 10 per cent of all healthy full-term babies, and in even more premature babies, this type of jaundice starts on the second or third day after birth, and disappears after about a week. It is particularly common in breast-fed babies, possibly because of very slight dehydration in the first few days of feeding.

ACTION

If jaundice seems to be getting worse, rather than better, or if it persists after two weeks, talk to your midwife or doctor right away. If the amount of bilirubin gets much too high, then there is a slight risk of brain damage.

USUAL TREATMENT

Bilirubin in the blood can be reduced by placing the baby under special fluorescent lights. This breaks it down into a harmless by-product that can then be removed from the body via the kidneys.

Very occasionally there may be other causes of jaundice, such as blood-group incompatibility between mother and child, or some rare liver abnormalities, and if jaundice does not seem to be fading, you should certainly ask for advice.

Kawasaki Disease

A rare childhood rash with potentially serious side-effects.

SYMPTOMS

This condition starts with a general red rash which tends to be worst over the knees and elbows. However, what makes the condition distinctive are the other signs and symptoms:

- High fever
- Swollen glands
- Bright red, cracked, sore lips
- A swollen tongue (with a surface like a large strawberry)

- Enlarged and readily visible blood vessels on the whites of the eyes, particularly around the iris (the brown, hazel or blue area)
- Swollen hands and feet
- Red palms and soles
- Peeling of the skin of the fingertips and ends of the toes (which usually is apparent after about a week)

ACTION

If you suspect that your child may be suffering from this condition, you should contact your doctor right away.

USUAL TREATMENT

While the majority of cases suffer no harmful effects at all, between 10 and 20 per cent of children with the condition can develop a heart problem. Prompt hospital treatment can dramatically reduce this risk. Your family doctor will ask a paediatrician to assess your child right away if this diagnosis is made. With early treatment there should be little or nothing in the way of long-term problems.

Kidney Disease

See also Urinary Tract Infections

Congenital and acquired kidney disorders can interfere with the removal of waste products from the body. The most common problem is an infection called pyelonephritis due to a urinary tract infection. A few children are born with only one kidney, while others have duplex kidneys that have two ureters, the tube that joins each kidney to the bladder.

SYMPTOMS

Symptoms of pyelonephritis include fever, pain on passing urine, lethargy, loss of appetite, vomiting, abdominal pain or pain around the sides of the trunk, and possibly a return to bedwetting. The symptoms of other kidney conditions can include fluid retention with puffiness around the eyes and ankles, and passing unusually small amounts of urine. Most congenital kidney problems do not cause any significant symptoms, and are often only discovered when some other problem, such as an infection, is being investigated.

ACTION

If you are concerned that your child is passing either too much or not enough urine, consult your doctor. Take a urine specimen collected in a clean bottle.

USUAL TREATMENT

Urinary tract infections are treated with antibiotics, but the management of other kidney problems depends entirely on cause.

Knock-Knees

See also Bow Legs

A condition in which the knees appear to be too close together, and which can make walking look clumsy.

SYMPTOMS

Young children are normally slightly wobbly on their legs when learning to walk. At this stage their legs can have the appearance of curving outwards slightly, often until the age of two years, when the legs gradually straighten out. By the age of three or four years the legs have usually straightened out, and then, as the child grows taller, the legs can look almost knock-kneed, with the knees appearing to turn inwards a little. To a certain degree it is absolutely normal for children to be slightly knock-kneed from the age of three until just before puberty.

ACTION

There is only cause for concern if your child seems much more knock-kneed than friends of the same age, if it is interfering with walking or running, and if it is not improving by the age of 10 to 11 in girls, or 12 to 13 in boys. If any of these are the case, then talk to your doctor.

USUAL TREATMENT

Most children with knock-knees do not need treatment or surgery. In the past, many different types of treatment were used, such as splinting or exercises. These treatments are no longer used because they were found to be of no benefit, particularly as the problem resolves spontaneously in 95 per cent of children.

Limping

See also Hip Problems ● Lyme Disease

A number of different conditions can cause a child to limp, with some being trivial and others much more important. Simple causes for limping include problems with footwear, a painful verruca, infected eczema affecting the foot, or a recent injection on that side.

SYMPTOMS

A child who limps tends to favour one leg, usually because something is making the other leg hurt. However, if your child limps and there is no obvious reason for the limp, then it is essential to have your child assessed by a doctor to exclude conditions such as Perthes' Disease (see Hip Problems, page 128).

ACTION

For minor aches and pains, you can try paracetamol and warm baths. If your child complains of pain causing limping that goes on for more than 24 hours with no obvious cause, seek medical advice. If the pain is severe, or if it is accompanied by a fever, then you should contact your doctor immediately.

USUAL TREATMENT

Treatment will depend on the cause of the limping. For minor conditions, such as irritable hip, rest will be all that is needed, but an x-ray may be taken to rule out more serious diagnoses. Hip pain that is diagnosed correctly and treated early should not cause long-term problems.

Lumps

See also Hernia ● Swollen Glands ● Throat Infections ● Umbilical Problems ● Warts

A lump on your child's body can be worrying but most skin lumps are caused by swollen lymph glands and are harmless. The lymph glands are located mainly in both the front and back of the neck, as well as in the armpits or groin. Lumps in the skin are also caused by boils, lipomas (or fatty swellings), sebaceous cysts (formed when a pore in the skin becomes blocked), warts and many other possibilities. Very rarely an isolated lump might possibly be a cancer.

SYMPTOMS

Lumps and swellings vary in size and consistency, depending on their cause and location. They may occasionally become hot and more swollen, or they may be filled with pus, as in the case of a boil.

ACTION

Most swollen glands will eventually disappear without treatment. However, if a swelling is hot, red and painful or grows larger, in comparison to its previous appearance, then seek your doctor's advice.

USUAL TREATMENT

Most swollen glands require no treatment at all. Sebaceous cysts and lipomas only need removing if they are unsightly.

Lyme Disease

This is a potentially serious infection caused by a tick bite. The ticks typically come from deer or mice, and occasionally from other animals and even humans. Incidentally, it is known as Lyme disease because it was first described in 1975 in the town of Old Lyme, Connecticut, USA.

SYMPTOMS

Children can develop Lyme disease after playing in long grass or other vegetation where animals might have been. The initial symptom is a skin reaction consisting of a ring that forms around the tick bite, and then gradually fades from the middle, although it can sometimes have a red centre. Although it sometimes looks similar to ringworm, the chief difference is that the appearance changes over a matter of a few days, whereas the changes of ringworm are much slower. As the bite may well have occurred in the scalp, these changes can remain invisible and unseen. About a month after the initial bite your child may develop symptoms very similar to having flu, with aching in the knees and other joints accompanied by a fever.

ACTION

It is essential to consult a doctor right away if you even vaguely suspect this condition, as untreated the symptoms can continue for months or even years, although they seem less severe. It can also have serious side-effects which can include damage to the eyes and heart.

USUAL TREATMENT

Once the diagnosis has been made and confirmed with blood tests, Lyme disease can be treated with antibiotics.

Masturbation

Self-stimulation of the sexual organs is extremely common, even at a very young age. As children discover different parts of their bodies, they will inevitably discover that handling the genitals can be pleasurable.

WHAT TO WATCH FOR

Up to the age of around five or six, both boys and girls are likely to masturbate frequently. Over this age, they realize this is not something to do in public, and the activity lessens.

ACTION

It is best to try to avoid paying too much attention and usually the child will discontinue masturbating. When your child is old enough to understand, you might point out that there are times and places when masturbation is not acceptable. You should consult your doctor if your child seems to masturbate compulsively, persists in public even after you have made it clear that this is not appropriate, or if your child seems in any other way upset or under strain, signs of which may include bed-wetting or soiling.

USUAL TREATMENT

Masturbation rarely needs any form of treatment. However, you might be more concerned if a child talks excessively about sexual matters and seems to have a knowledge inappropriate for his or her age. This could raise the possibility either of some form of abuse, or that the child has been exposed to inappropriate scenes such as pornographic videos. If you have any concerns in this area, then talk to your doctor. It is probably worth having a consultation with the doctor without your child first.

Measles

This used to be a very common infectious illness, but, thanks to immunization, it has now become rare in the UK, although in certain countries world-wide it continues to be very serious and potentially fatal. Some children who have been immunized against measles may develop a milder version of the condition.

SYMPTOMS

A blotchy, red rash usually starts on the child's face, particularly behind the ears. It then spreads over the trunk, the arms and the legs. The child tends to have a high temperature, a fierce barking cough and red or sticky eyes. In the first couple of days he or she may have white spots inside the mouth.

ACTION

The incubation period is between 7 and 18 days, and the condition is infectious from just before the illness starts until four days after the rash appears. Because the disease is notifiable (which means that your doctor has to tell your local health authority so that they can monitor the immunization system), and because it may not be measles, you should certainly consult your doctor if you suspect this condition. Complications include earache and a persistent cough. The most serious, but rare, complication is encephalitis, inflammation affecting the brain. The symptoms of this are headache, neck ache or possibly backache, and in later stages possibly fits. Call your doctor at once if your child has these symptoms.

USUAL TREATMENT

Keep your child cool, give paracetamol and lots to drink. Some children may develop a middle ear or chest infection which may require an antibiotic.

Meningitis

See also Headache ● Migraine

An infection that affects the meninges, which are the membranes that surround the brain and the spinal cord. There are two types of meningitis: the milder viral form and the very serious bacterial infection, meningococcal meningitis. As well as being potentially fatal, it can also leave disabilities, such as deafness, epilepsy or cerebral palsy. However, despite the alarming seriousness of the illness, and the publicity it gets, meningitis is still a relatively rare condition.

SYMPTOMS

BACTERIAL MENINGITIS
The symptoms of bacterial meningitis may include:

● Fever

● Strong headache

● Neck stiffness

● Aversion to bright light

● Drowsiness

● Distress on handling

● Nausea

● Vomiting or diarrhoea

● Tense or bulging fontanelle (the 'soft spot' in the skull) – in babies

● A widespread, purple bruise-like rash that does not fade when a glass tumbler is pressed against it (see pages 160–2, and illustration between pages 128 and 129)

● A baby may be off her feed

A stiff neck or a headache can be a sign of meningitis. Looking out for symptoms is vitally important, but the vast majority of children who complain of a stiff neck or headache do not have meningitis, but are instead suffering from something much less serious. However, it is certainly worth checking every time with your doctor.

To check to see if your toddler's neck is stiff, ask him to lie down and get him to look at his

Meningitis

SYMPTOMS *continued*

tummy button. If your child can bend the head slightly forward, meningitis is extremely unlikely. Ask an older child to put his or her chin onto the chest.

VIRAL MENINGITIS
The symptoms of viral meningitis are much less alarming and are similar to flu, with aching joints, a fever and perhaps a headache.

ACTION

Your child will usually have other symptoms before the headache starts. These may be as mild as a sore throat and fever. If your child then develops severe headache and vomiting, he or she should be seen urgently by a doctor. It's important to note that a rash may not always be present. Call your GP or go immediately to your local Accident and Emergency department. If in doubt, phone 999.

USUAL TREATMENT

BACTERIAL MENINGITIS
The sooner that a child with meningitis can be given intravenous penicillin, the better the outcome. Even though meningitis is still rare, it is still important to make contact with a doctor urgently if you strongly suspect that your child may have this condition. Going to the doctor or local hospital Accident and Emergency department may be quicker than waiting for a home visit. Diagnosis is made by testing fluid drawn from the spinal cord using a procedure called a lumbar puncture. This can be a very distressing procedure for parents of young children, and it may be best if you are not present while it is done.

VIRAL MENINGITIS
Viral meningitis will usually clear up in one to two weeks without any treatment apart from paracetamol for the aches and fever.

Molluscum Contagiosum

See also Warts

This common condition produces crops of small swellings in the skin. They are caused by a virus growing in the surface layers of the skin and are similar to tiny warts.

SYMPTOMS

The smooth, pearly white or skin-coloured shiny spots are usually between 3 and 8 mm in diameter, have a small dimple in the centre and may be filled with fluid. They can occur almost anywhere on the body, but are most common on the trunk or the buttocks. The spots are not usually itchy.

ACTION

This condition is not dangerous, and the spots are harmless. See your doctor if you aren't sure of the diagnosis.

USUAL TREATMENT

The spots will eventually disappear without treatment. If they are numerous, embarrassing or unsightly, or if they are worrying your child, your doctor may scratch the top of them and apply a chemical known as phenol. Some doctors will also use cryotherapy, which involves freezing the spots with liquid nitrogen, although this can be uncomfortable. Despite the name, molluscum contagiosum is not particularly contagious. Nevertheless it would still be wise for other children to avoid direct contact with the actual spots.

Mumps

See also Lumps ● Vaccination

A viral infection causing swelling of the salivary glands. Mumps is now quite rare, since the introduction of the MMR (measles, mumps and rubella) vaccine.

SYMPTOMS

Usually there is marked and often painful swelling of the salivary glands, found at the angle of the jaw just in front of and below the ear lobes. One or both sides of the neck can be affected. In general, the swelling lasts for a few days. Your child will also have a temperature, and boys may develop discomfort in the testicles. Rarely, a type of meningitis may accompany the infection.

ACTION

Consult your doctor to have the diagnosis confirmed. If your child develops a severe headache or testicular pain, seek medical help right away.

USUAL TREATMENT

No treatment is needed as the infection will clear within a few days. Give your child paracetamol and offer bland foods and plenty to drink. Tasty foods cause more saliva to be produced and this can be painful. Your child is infectious from about one week before the symptoms appear to approximately two weeks after the illness is apparent.

Muscular Dystrophy

An inherited disorder which causes slow but progressive degeneration of muscle fibres, resulting in weakness and disability. Some forms appear at birth, while others may not become apparent until after the age of 50. They are all rare. The most common is Duchenne muscular dystrophy, an inherited disorder that only affects boys.

SYMPTOMS

Duchenne dystrophy is rarely diagnosed before the age of three years, but then tends to progress rapidly. Children with the condition are slow to sit up and walk, and a quarter will have some form of mental handicap.

Mobility gradually deteriorates and walking becomes impossible by the age of 12. Because the cardiac muscles are also weakened, there is also the risk of persistent chest infection.

ACTION

If you are concerned about your child's muscular development, or believe that he or she is slow in walking or learning other motor skills, then talk to your health visitor or GP. Your child may then be referred to a specialist for blood tests, an EMG (electromyogram) – which tests electrical activity in the muscles – and a muscle biopsy.

USUAL TREATMENT

While there is no effective treatment, it is important for children with this condition to keep as active as possible. A paediatric physiotherapist will advise and assist you. It is also important to keep your child from becoming overweight. Parents and siblings of an affected child will also be offered genetic counselling to explain any future risks.

Nappy Rash

See also Fungal Infections

A rash affecting the skin on a baby's bottom in the area normally covered by a nappy. There are several causes: urine and faeces being left in contact with the skin for a period of time, the fungal infection thrush or occasionally a reaction to chemicals in soap powder if terry nappies are being used.

SYMPTOMS

Nappy rash can vary from very mild redness, to an inflamed, very sore-looking skin extending over the whole of the baby's bottom.

In nappy rash caused by thrush, there can be a white discharge and areas of redness away from the main rash.

ACTION

Fungus infections thrive on warmth and moisture so the more the area is exposed to the air, the less likely the rash is to develop and spread; leaving nappies off from time to time is a good idea. Consult a doctor if the rash looks very inflamed or there are pimples and blisters. Zinc oxide or barrier creams can also help to prevent the rash. Try to wash your baby's bottom every two to three hours and use a one-way disposable nappy liner.

USUAL TREATMENT

Anti-fungal creams such as Canesten and keeping the napkin area clean and dry are the mainstays of treatment.

Neck Pain

See also Meningitis ● Sore Throat

While pain in the neck often causes parents to worry about meningitis, the cause is far more likely to be a harmless muscular condition. It is very common for children to develop a spasm in one side of the neck, either after a minor injury, or on waking up in the morning. This is called a 'wry neck'.

SYMPTOMS

Neck pain is best checked by asking the child to put his or her chin on each shoulder in turn. In wry neck this will be possible on one side, but not on the other. Moving the chin onto the chest is usually painless, and your child will be well in every other way.

Children sometimes complain of neck discomfort if they have swollen glands which result from a throat infection. This swelling will typically be on just one side. In meningitis (see page 146), the stiffness prevents the child from bending the head forward.

ACTION

One of the most effective treatments is either a warm hot water bottle held onto the area of spasm for a couple of minutes every hour (but make sure it is not too hot), or alternatively use an ice pack. You can also use a small bag of frozen peas or sweetcorn wrapped in a tea towel. Gently encourage your child to move the neck. Give paracetamol or ibuprofen to relieve any pain.

USUAL TREATMENT

If the discomfort is severe, or lasts more than 24 hours, see your doctor who might need to arrange physiotherapy.

Nightmares and Night Terrors

Disturbances of sleep which usually appear to be distressing for the child.

WHAT TO WATCH FOR

Nightmares are dreams about something frightening. They are more likely to occur if your child is anxious or worried. They may be aggravated by colds and nasal congestion. Night terrors typically occur between two and six years of age and are different from nightmares in that they do not occur during the dreaming phase of sleep. This means that the child never has any recollection of what has happened, even though he or she may be found screaming, frequently sitting up and staring, oblivious to anyone in the room. Night terrors are not a sign of emotional problems – they seem to just happen.

ACTION

If your child is having a nightmare, it will do no harm if you gently wake him or her. However, it's almost impossible to get through to a child who is having a night terror; you may want to sit in the room for your own peace of mind.

If your child is having nightmares, keep an eye on his or her games and drawings, as the cause of the worries may become apparent. It may then just be a matter of talking the problem through and offering gentle reassurance.

USUAL TREATMENT

If a child is having night terrors night after night, they probably occur at exactly the same time. Set your alarm for 10 minutes before the usual time and go in and gently wake your child who will then drift back to sleep and the terror won't happen. This is a simple but highly effective technique.

Non-accidental Injury

See also Bruising ● Bullying

This is the deliberate physical abuse of children.

WHAT TO WATCH FOR

The great majority of the injuries that happen to children are accidents. However, deliberate injury may occasionally occur, and these injuries are usually caused by family members or other care-givers. If you are concerned that you have harmed your child, or feel that you might do so, then please talk to your GP or health visitor right away. Many parents become extremely stressed, particularly with constantly crying children, but help really is available.

The typical clues of someone having harmed your child include injuries which are not consistent with the story of what happened, a delay in reporting injuries, inconsistent stories from people who saw what took place, or recurrent injuries.

ACTION

If you are concerned that your child has been in any way harmed deliberately, then you should consult your doctor as soon as is practical. It may well be that there is an innocent explanation but, if a carer, such as a child minder, is causing harm to your child, then the problem is too important to ignore.

USUAL TREATMENT

It there is cause for concern, your doctor or health visitor will notify an expert such as a social worker who will co-ordinate investigation and further action. If necessary, your child will be assessed by a paediatrician.

Nosebleeds

See also Clotting Disorders ● Foreign Bodies

Bleeding can come from the nose, usually when the small blood vessels on the inner surface of the nose break or are broken. Nosebleeds can be very dramatic but are hardly ever serious.

SYMPTOMS

Bleeding usually occurs from just one side of the nose and blood can also drain into the back of the throat, sometimes making it appear that a child is coughing up blood. Perhaps the most common cause of a nosebleed is an inserted finger – picking the nose is a common childhood habit. Other causes include blowing the nose very hard, violent sneezing or an allergic reaction.

ACTION

Small nosebleeds are very common and not dangerous. Agitation makes bleeding worse, so try to calm your child down if he seems worried. If the nosebleed is severe, sit your child up and provide a bowl he or she can lean over. Squeeze the nose firmly for five minutes. If you have any ice cubes, put a couple in a polythene bag and then squeeze the nose between them. Never try to insert anything up the nose, not even cotton wool.

USUAL TREATMENT

If the bleeding persists for more than half an hour, or if your child gets repeated nosebleeds, consult your doctor.

Osgood-Schlatter Disease

See also Limping

Painful knees caused by inflammation at the point where the tendon that holds the kneecap is attached to the upper tibia, one of the bones in the lower leg.

SYMPTOMS

Your child will complain of pain in one knee, particularly on exercising. You may notice a swelling of the prominent area of bone on the front of the upper tibia. This condition can cause considerable discomfort on running, or other activities such as going up and down stairs.

ACTION

Painful knees, caused by whatever condition, are not particularly common in small children, so if your child complains repeatedly that his or her knees hurt you should always seek medical advice. The doctor will examine the knee joints, paying particular attention to the kneecaps. Sometimes painful knees result from problems with the hips, so your doctor will probably examine these joints too.

USUAL TREATMENT

Osgood-Schlatter disease is not serious and almost always recovers fully in time without treatment. If it is painful, then rest can help very considerably. Schools may ask for confirmation from your doctor that your child should avoid games and sports.

Pain

See also The Home Medicine Chest ● Tummy Ache

There are many possible causes of pain, including injury, infection and inflammation.

WHAT TO WATCH FOR

Any pain has two separate components, the physical (in the body) and the psychological (in the mind). Fear, apprehension and anxiety can greatly worsen pain, and doctors and parents are well aware that much pain can be reduced by a calm and reassuring manner. While some pains – such as Monday morning pre-school tummy aches – are clearly entirely psychological, no recurrent pain should be blamed on psychological causes until a doctor has examined and assessed your child.

ACTION

Be concerned about any pain that lasts for more than six hours or wakes your child. If you know the cause, pain-relieving medication usually helps. If the cause is not obvious, consult a doctor who will ask a number of questions such as what type of pain is it, where does it spread to, does anything make it worse, does anything make it better, is the child otherwise well? Give thought to these in advance and encourage your child to tell the doctor. If your child is screaming in pain, contact your doctor or go to the local Accident and Emergency department at once.

USUAL TREATMENT

For most children painkillers such as paracetamol or ibuprofen will be very helpful. Warmth and gentle massage may also help.

Pet-related Problems

While pets may be cuddly and lovable, they can also pass on infections and parasites. A number of basic hygiene precautions should be followed to avoid illness and discomfort.

SYMPTOMS

Apart from allergies to pets, which cause symptoms such as itching, wheezing or a runny nose, and itchy bites from their fleas, there are two important infections to watch for:

Toxocariosis is an infestation with a small roundworm called *Toxocara canis*. This organism lives in the dog's digestive tract. Children who play on soil contaminated with dogs' faeces can accidentally pass the worm's eggs from their hands into their mouths. Once in the child's intestines, these worms hatch into larvae which can cause a number of serious conditions such as allergies, pneumonia, fits or loss of vision.

Toxoplasmosis is caused by an organism found in cat faeces. Its most severe effects are on the unborn foetus, but it can cause a feverish illness and visual problems in both children and adults.

ACTION

If you think your child is infected, see your doctor. Clean up any pet faeces in the garden. Use a pooper scooper if your dog defecates in a public place. Make sure your children wash their hands after playing outside and always before eating.

USUAL TREATMENT

The most important treatment is prevention, so worm and deflea your pets. Your child might need blood tests, and might be referred to a paediatrician.

Pyloric Stenosis

See also Vomiting

Thickening of the pylorus, the strong muscular valve found where the stomach empties into the duodenum, or small intestine, is the most significant cause of forceful vomiting in babies. The stomach muscle tightens in an attempt to force the milk past the blockage and, since this cannot happen, the stomach contents are instead pushed forcefully up through the oesophagus and out through the mouth.

SYMPTOMS

Symptoms usually appear between two and six weeks of age, and babies with this condition are typically hungry, crying to be fed almost immediately after sicking up milk-coloured vomit. Hunger results from lack of food being able to pass into the intestine for normal absorption. Babies with this condition are constipated, and fail to gain weight.

ACTION

Occasional projectile vomiting is not uncommon, but if it happens repeatedly you should certainly consult a doctor.

USUAL TREATMENT

Your baby will be immediately referred for assessment by a paediatrician. An ultrasound scan will be used to confirm if the condition is present. If it is confirmed, a small operation will be carried out to divide the thickened muscle fibres around the pylorus, so freeing up the outlet from the stomach.

Rashes

See also Allergy ● Chickenpox ● Cold Sores ● Eczema
● Fifth Disease ● Hand, Foot and Mouth Disease
● Impetigo ● Kawasaki Disease ● Lyme Disease
● Measles ● Molluscum Contagiosum ● Ringworm
● Roseola Infantum ● Rubella ● Scabies ● Scarlet Fever
● Urticaria ● See illustrations between pages 128 and 129

Rashes are very common and have many different possible
causes. Parents want to know what each rash is, what causes it,
whether it is serious, whether it is infectious, and what they
should do about it. By using a series of simple questions and
answers, these pages should guide you to the likely cause of
your child's rash. However, it is impossible to cover every
possible cause of childhood rashes here so this section covers
the most common. As always, if you are in the least doubt, then
you should consult your doctor.

DIAGNOSING RASHES

Most medical diagnoses are
reached by a process that is very
similar to detective work. The
doctor asks a number of
questions, looks at a number of
clues, tries to piece all the
information together, and
finally arrives at an answer.
When unravelling the cause of a
rash you can do the same.
Sometimes the answer will be
obvious – a nettle rash in a child
who has just walked through a
nettle bed is an obvious example
– but more often than not, you
will have to piece various clues
together. Inevitably, not every
rash can be diagnosed simply,
but at the very least this guide
can point you in the right
direction. Look in turn at the
questions listed below: they will
guide you towards a possible
diagnosis. If you can only

DIAGNOSING RASHES *continued*

answer yes to one question, then you will probably have a number of possibilities; but if you answer yes to two or more questions, the diagnosis will become much more obvious. For instance, if you answer yes to 'Does the rash itch?', and 'Is it worse on the front of the elbows or back of the knees?', but you answer no to 'Does your child have a temperature?' and 'Is your child unwell?', then the likely diagnosis will be eczema. Incidentally, when diagnosing a rash it really is important to undress your child completely and look at the skin in all parts of the body; otherwise you may find yourself jumping to unjustified conclusions.

QUESTIONS TO ASK

Does your child have a temperature with the rash?
Yes: possible causes include chickenpox, measles, roseola infantum, rubella or scarlet fever

Has your child recently had any injections?
Yes: a rash may occur about a week after the MMR (measles, mumps and rubella) vaccination

Has the rash been present for more than a couple of weeks, or does it keep coming back?
Yes: causes include eczema or fungal rashes

If there is no temperature, does the rash itch?
Yes: likely causes are eczema or urticaria

Is the rash confined to one part of the body?
Yes: possible causes include contact eczema (dermatitis) or impetigo

Is the scalp dry, flaky or thickened?
Yes: possible causes include dandruff, fungal infections or seborrhoeic dermatitis (cradle cap)

Rashes

Are the feet affected mainly, with a scaly rash on the toes or the ball of the foot?
Yes: likely causes include athlete's foot or eczema

Does your child also have a cough?
Yes: a possible cause is measles. If the rash is confined to the area around the eyes, this may come from tiny burst blood vessels from the strain of coughing and is harmless.

What does the rash look like?
a) Dry, red, itchy skin: likely cause is eczema
b) Distinct, dry and scaly separate patches: possible causes include eczema or ringworm

Is the rash flat and under the skin?
Yes: likely causes include allergic reactions, fifth disease, Kawasaki disease, measles, rubella, roseola or scarlet fever

Does the rash consist of flat pink or red spots, with normal skin in between?
Yes: possible causes include a drug reaction or viral infection

Is the rash mainly in the form of blisters?
Yes: likely to be chickenpox (starts as red spots), cold sores, hand, foot and mouth disease, impetigo or insect bites.

Is there only one yellow and crusty blister, possibly infected?
Yes: possible causes include cold sores or impetigo

Are the blisters mainly on the hands, feet, and mouth?
Yes: likely to be hand, foot and mouth disease

Is the rash raised, but without blisters?
Yes: likely causes include scabies or urticaria

Are there tiny white waxy bumps on the skin, often in clusters?
Yes: probable cause is molluscum contagiosum

Does the rash have one or more rings, possibly with a clear centre?
Yes: possible causes include Lyme disease or ringworm

Ringworm

Ringworm is a common fungus infection of the skin.

SYMPTOMS

Don't be alarmed by the name – there's no worm involved. The 'ring' describes the shape of the rash, and the 'worm' refers to the appearance of the edge of the rash, which is raised and looks like a curled-up worm lying on the skin. Ringworm usually causes one or more circular patches of raised red skin, with scaly edges and a clear centre. The circle grows very slowly and the condition can persist for a long time. The rash can occur anywhere on the skin, including the scalp, and can cause an itchy form of dandruff, and dandruff in any child under age 10 should make you suspect ringworm.

ACTION

If you suspect ringworm, consult your doctor. He or she may confirm the diagnosis, or may gently scrape away a few small flakes of skin to be sent off to the laboratory for examination under a microscope to identify the fungus involved.

USUAL TREATMENT

An anti-fungal cream such as clotrimazole (Canesten) is usually very effective. If this is not, consult your doctor again who may prescribe stronger creams or medication to be taken by mouth. Ringworm is also quite easily passed from child to child, and flourishes in warm, humid conditions. Transmission is by direct contact, so keep a dressing on the rash if it is on an exposed part of the body and your child is going to school. School medical authorities may not admit the child back to school until treatment has started.

Roseola Infantum

See also Convulsions

A common but not well-known viral infection which causes a fever and rash.

SYMPTOMS

Roseola infantum mainly occurs between six months and two years of age, and starts with a high fever, possibly accompanied by a sore throat. The fever goes on for three or four days, and as the child's temperature settles back to normal, a non-itchy, reddish rash appears all over the body (see page 160). The rash lasts for a couple of days and then gradually fades away. One of the most typical features of the illness is that your child will feel much better when the rash appears and her temperature drops.

ACTION

If you are worried, then seek advice, if only to have the diagnosis confirmed. If your child's temperature rises sharply, try to keep your child cool by sponging with tepid water to reduce the risk of febrile convulsion (which occasionally happens with this condition because of the high fever). Call your doctor if the fever continues to rise or if your child has a convulsion.

USUAL TREATMENT

Because roseola infantum is caused by a virus, antibiotics do not help. The illness rarely needs any treatment other than paracetamol or ibuprofen for the fever and certainly isn't infectious enough to keep your child away from other children.

Rubella

Also known as German measles, rubella is a virus which, thanks to vaccination, is becoming much less common, but cases do still occur occasionally.

SYMPTOMS

The main symptom is a pinky-red rash (see pages 160–2, and illustration between pages 128 and 129) that starts on the face, spreads to the trunk and then to the arms and legs. Your child will also have swollen glands behind the ears.

ACTION

See your doctor to have the diagnosis confirmed. The condition is relatively mild and harmless. However, if it affects pregnant women, it can cause major problems for unborn children, leading to blindness, deafness, heart disease and other problems. For this reason your child should be kept at home. The majority of women will be fine, as they will already be immune, but it is essential that they are checked by a doctor or midwife if exposed to your child.

USUAL TREATMENT

Rubella rarely needs treatment, other than paracetamol, and almost never causes any complications, although older girls occasionally have aching joints. School medical advisers usually suggest that a child with rubella should stay off school for a week after the onset of the rash.

Scabies

An infestation by mites causing intense itching and a rash.

SYMPTOMS

The scabies mite burrows under the skin, especially in the webs of skin between the fingers and the toes, the back of the hands, the wrists, the palms and the abdomen. The head and neck are sometimes affected in babies. The rash (see pages 160–2, and illustration between pages 128 and 129), which is very infectious and intensely itchy (especially at night), is caused by an allergy to the mite, its eggs and the larvae. The itching may begin a couple of days before the actual rash breaks out. Symptoms can take up to a month to develop, so a child can pass the mite on before anyone is aware of the infection. The mite can be spread by close physical contact, and in particular sharing of beds or of items of clothing. It can only live for up to four days away from human skin, so fabrics that have not had contact with human skin for more than four days will not harbour live mites.

ACTION

If you suspect scabies, contact your doctor who will prescribe a suitable lotion. Two or more preparations might be needed before a complete cure is achieved.

USUAL TREATMENT

It is essential to apply the lotion to the whole body, especially to the webs of the fingers and toes and under the fingernails. In children under two, apply the treatment to the scalp, neck, face and ears. In older children and adults, just apply the lotion up to the neck. It is important to treat the whole family. Calamine lotion, a hydrocortisone cream such as Eurax or even oral antihistamines will help to control the itching.

Scalp Problems

See also Cradle Cap ● Eczema ● Head Lice

The scalp may be affected by almost any skin condition such as eczema, as well as by infestations such as head lice.

SYMPTOMS

The most common cause of an itchy scalp are head lice, dandruff, cradle cap and eczema. It is important to make a definite diagnosis, as treating eczema with head lice treatment will obviously make the situation much worse, and vice versa. Dandruff is usually caused by a condition known as seborrhoeic dermatitis, which causes flakes of dead skin to be shed from the scalp surface.

ACTION

Examine your child's scalp for head lice, and look at the skin on your child's neck, trunk, and back to see if there is any evidence of eczema. Most dandruff can be treated initially with a good anti-dandruff shampoo, but check with the pharmacist that it's safe for children. If you find plaques of thickened skin, then consult your doctor for advice as these might be a sign of eczema or cradle cap, which need different types of treatment.

USUAL TREATMENT

If the diagnosis is confirmed as seborrhoeic dermatitis, your doctor may prescribe an anti-fungal shampoo such as Nizoral. Do not use these medicated shampoos on other children without medical advice. Scalp eczema may require treatment with a form of steroid lotion.

Scarlet Fever

See also Sore Throat

An infection caused by a bacteria known as streptococcus, which causes a severe sore throat and a bright red rash.

SYMPTOMS

Scarlet fever (or scarlatina) is most common before the teenage years. It usually starts with a severe sore throat and a rash of tiny spots that can feel like sandpaper and turn pale when pressed firmly. The rash begins on the neck and the chest, and then spreads to the whole of the body, tending to be worse along skin folds, in the groin or armpit for example. Some children may be very ill with a high fever, vomiting, a red and flushed face but a pale area around the mouth, a white-coated tongue with red patches known as a strawberry tongue, and even peeling of the skin.

ACTION

Antibiotics are always needed so consult your GP. Also, give plenty of fluids, paracetamol and lots of sympathy. The disease is infectious until the sufferer has been on an antibiotic for 48 hours.

USUAL TREATMENT

Scarlet fever is treated with antibiotics, usually penicillin, because it carries a small risk of complications such as ear infections, inflammation of the kidneys (nephritis) or rheumatic fever. The antibiotics probably do not make much of a difference to the scarlet fever itself, but they certainly help to prevent these potentially serious complications.

School Phobia

See also Bullying ● Depression

A fear of attending school that may cause a child to 'invent' illness in order to miss classes on a frequent basis.

WHAT TO WATCH FOR

Your child may state quite openly that he or she does not want to go to school, and may even tell you why. However, it is just as likely that the situation will become apparent through repeated physical illnesses on school days. Conditions such as nausea, headaches or tummy aches may be particularly difficult to deal with as it may be quite impossible at first to tell if the pain is genuine or not. If you are in doubt, it is important to get your child checked by a doctor rather than jumping to conclusions.

The main clue that school is the cause of a symptom comes if the problem clears up at weekends and during school holidays. There are two main causes of school phobias:

● Fear of something that might happen at school

● Separation anxiety: your child is worried about what might happen at home while he or she is away at school

In addition, children may become anxious about school if they have a problem with seeing or hearing in class. A child who cannot properly see or hear what is going on can feel very frightened and anxious, and may be too embarrassed or confused to tell anyone about it.

ACTION

Once you feel certain that the problem is school phobia, it is important to find out the cause. Talk to teachers to see how your child gets on at school and to find out if there is a problem with bullying or a relationship with a teacher or friend that may

School Phobia

ACTION *continued*

be causing difficulties. A major step in managing the problem may lie in realizing that the focus of the concern may not be the school itself, but is actually in the home. If there has been a problem at home, such as a bereavement or marital problems, then this may be the source of any separation anxiety your child is exhibiting. If your child is terrified that you will die or disappear the moment he or she lets you out of sight, then going to school becomes a worrying event.

USUAL TREATMENT

It is important that your child realizes that school is not an optional activity. Agree on a day for a return to school and stick to it. This may be very upsetting for you as a parent, particularly if your child pleads with you to let him or her stay at home, but getting your child back to school can boost self-confidence and is a major step in sorting out the problem in the long term.

The longer the child stays away from school, the bigger the hurdle becomes of having to return. Parents often feel secretly flattered that their child wants to spend so much time with them, rather than going to school, but this really is not an option.

If the problem is separation anxiety, your child needs to develop confidence in being away from you without anything dreadful happening. Reassure your child again and again that you will be there when he or she returns. A short stay away, overnight perhaps, with family or friends nearby can be an excellent first step toward resolving problems.

If the problem persists, despite your best efforts and those of the school, consult your GP who may refer your child to a child psychologist or family centre for extra help in dealing with any concerns you or your child might have.

Scoliosis

A deformity of the spine which results in its being bent over towards one side, appearing to have an S shape rather than being straight. It is much more common in girls than boys.

SYMPTOMS

Scoliosis may be present at birth, or result from an injury. It gradually gets worse until growth finally stops at the end of adolescence, with deterioration happening particularly at times of growth spurts. Parents frequently do not notice this condition, which is often picked up in medical examinations. The main symptoms are that one shoulder blade appears much higher than the other, and the child's posture makes one side of the rib cage appear more prominent. The way to see whether the spine is genuinely curved is to look at the spine as your child bends over to touch her toes.

ACTION

If you suspect that your child has scoliosis, go to your GP who may arrange an x-ray to confirm the diagnosis. Minor degrees of scoliosis need no treatment, but it is likely that your child will be referred for a specialist opinion and regular monitoring.

USUAL TREATMENT

Early diagnosis is necessary to prevent deformity and lung problems. Physiotherapy may be of help and, in more severe forms of scoliosis, treatment may be needed. This can include the use of a brace. In very severe cases, spinal surgery may be needed in order to fuse the vertebrae together so that they stay in a straight line.

Shingles

See also Chickenpox

A painful skin rash caused by the chickenpox virus.

SYMPTOMS

If your child has had chickenpox, the virus (herpes zoster) will then hibernate in the root of any of the main nerves that come out of the spine. The virus can be re-activated spontaneously or if the patient is run down, and this produces a chickenpox-like, extremely painful, blistering rash in the area of the skin that the nerve in question goes to. Since the nerves run to specific areas of skin, the rash only appears in the area reached by the affected nerve. This can be anywhere on the face, trunk or limbs but will only ever affect one side of the body at a time and will only be in a relatively small area on that side.

ACTION

Give painkillers and consult your doctor. If your child is on steroid treatment or immunosuppressant therapy for another illness, contact your doctor immediately, as in these cases shingles can become a dangerous condition.

USUAL TREATMENT

Most doctors will prescribe an anti-viral drug such as acyclovir, which will shorten the attack. Paracetamol will help with pain relief, and calamine lotion will help to reduce the itching. It is possible to catch chickenpox from shingles, so your child should not mix with others who might be at risk for the first few days. Rest helps speed recovery.

Sibling Rivalry

See also Terrible Twos

There can also be intense competition between your children; this is known as sibling rivalry.

WHAT TO WATCH FOR

Sibling rivalry is particularly likely to occur at times of important events such as the birth of a new baby brother or sister. The older child may well have been the focus of attention for all his or her life, and can feel extremely rejected by the new arrival. However, younger children can also be jealous of the privileges they see their older siblings being granted. Rivalry tends to be at its worst when one of the children is two or three years old.

ACTION

Always avoid comparing one child unfavourably with another: all your children are individuals.

Encourage your children to play together as much as possible, and to share their belongings.

USUAL TREATMENT

You will at times treat the older child differently to the younger one – it would be absurd not to. Try to give each child a slot of your time that is theirs, and theirs alone. Telling an older child, 'You're still my baby, too', can be greatly reassuring. If, despite trying all this, you are still struggling with the problem, ask your health visitor for advice.

Sleep Problems

See also Nightmares and Night Terrors ● Crying

Repeated sleepless or broken nights are one of the biggest sources of stress for parents of young children. Many babies and toddlers sleep less than the accepted norm, but as long as they are happy during their waking hours and do not seem unwell, they do not need medical attention.

WHAT TO WATCH FOR

Four out of 10 children aged between six months and five years are reported to have some sleep problems. This is not helped by the advice parents may read saying things like 'the average four-year-old should sleep for ten hours each night.' This sort of statement is fine if your child does sleep, but what if he doesn't? Parents worry that either there is something wrong with their child or with the way they are bringing him up. In fact, parents are frequently led towards entirely unrealistic expectations. However, despite this, there are three main types of childhood sleep problem:

● The child who won't go to sleep at night

● The child who wakes repeatedly

● The child who wakes early

It is important to realize that there is only a problem if you have a problem. If your child wakes 20 times a night and it doesn't bother you, then you haven't got a problem. Doctors or health visitors assessing the situation are rarely concerned about how children sleep, but rather about how any sleep disturbance the child may have affects the parents.

ACTION

There are several things you can do to try to improve sleep problems:

- Try to introduce a regular bedtime routine. The actual shape of the routine is entirely up to you, but it could include a bath, story and cuddle. Using the same routine every night will encourage your child to settle down more readily.

- Don't feel guilty if your child has a sleep problem. There is no evidence that parents cause children to wake, though you can learn ways of coping better if they do.

- Don't rush in if you hear your child stir in the night. Children tend to wake more frequently than adults anyway, and will often cry out, roll over and go back to sleep again. If from the start you rush in, put the light on, and check that your child is all right, then he or she will almost certainly wake completely.

- Don't use cough medicines or antihistamines as sedatives. They do not work, are potentially dangerous and will leave your child miserable the next day.

- Try not to feed a baby to sleep. If a baby is always fed to sleep, he learns that he needs something in his mouth to settle, so if he wakes he is likely to cry until given a bottle or breast. By gently waking a baby at the end of a feed and then lying him down, he will learn to be able to sleep without the feed continuing and so will be less likely to cry out on waking.

USUAL TREATMENT

If you simply aren't winning with sleep problems, talk to your health visitor or doctor. The main technique that health visitors and doctors now use is a form of behavioural therapy, and this can help many different types of sleep problem. Behavioural therapy teaches children new ways of acting in certain situations. As an example, consider the child who won't go to sleep alone in the

Sleep Problems

evening. Say goodnight to your child, then leave the room. If your child won't settle, wait for five minutes before you go back in, however loud the crying. Then go in, briefly reassure your child, and leave again. Do not give a drink or a cuddle. This time, wait 10 minutes before you go back in. Again, make your visit brief, and leave the room. Now wait 15 minutes before you go back. The next time, leave it 20 minutes, and so on.

During one of these waits outside the room, your child will go quiet. If this happens do not go back in. Your child has learnt to go to sleep without you. The next night may well be much easier. Most children will be sleeping well in about a week.

This method is completely different from just leaving your child to cry, and is much less stressful for parents. By returning, you are reassuring yourself that all is well, but the child is learning that crying brings no other reward. However, don't weaken and offer a cuddle after the fourth return to the room, or your child will have learnt that persistent crying pays. Make sure you use a clock or watch to time the intervals. A minute can seem like an hour when listening to a screaming child.

Try to appear relaxed and friendly if you possibly can. This can be difficult if your child has been screaming for an hour, and any normal parent will feel his or her irritation level rising rapidly, but if you can be kind and firm you are far more likely to succeed. If you don't seem to be getting anywhere, leave it for a week and then try the behavioural therapy approach again. Inform neighbours so they understand why your child will be crying longer for a few days.

Sleepwalking

A condition in which a child is completely asleep yet is able to walk and even climb stairs and manoeuvre through doors.

WHAT TO WATCH FOR

Around 15 per cent of children have sleepwalked at least once, though it is most common after the age of five years. A typical sleepwalking episode consists of the child suddenly sitting bolt upright in bed, eyes open but unseeing. He gets up, may open cupboards or doors as if looking for something, and moves with rather clumsy movements. Attempts to talk to a sleepwalking child will be met with little more than grunts. The child eventually goes back to bed, falls back to normal sleep, and in the morning will remember nothing of what has happened.

ACTION

Occasional sleepwalking is not a problem, as long as your child cannot injure him- or herself. It is not true that sleepwalkers cannot injure themselves, so apply some basic protective measures, such as locking large bedroom windows or blocking off the stairs.

USUAL TREATMENT

There is some evidence that a relaxing bedtime routine may help lessen the incidence of sleepwalking. Don't worry if your child sleepwalks only occasionally but, if it is a regular occurrence and is causing problems, consult your doctor. If sleepwalking is a major problem, sleeping medication may help to prevent it.

Interestingly, sleepwalking does not occur during the dreaming phase of sleep, which means that your child is not acting out activities that he or she is dreaming about. This is also the reason why he or she does not remember the episode later on.

Snoring

See also Allergy ● Hayfever

Noisy breathing through the nose that occurs during sleep.

SYMPTOMS

As well as the noise of snoring, which may disturb the sleep of other family members, children who snore may breathe through the mouth during the day because the nasal airways are blocked. This is common in the first four or five years due to a combination of factors, mainly because the tonsils and the adenoids (glandular swellings found at the back of the nasal passages) are at their largest. Allergic conditions that aggravate nasal congestion can worsen the problem. Snoring by itself is not a cause for concern unless it is disturbing your child's sleep.

ACTION

Don't sew a cork into the back of the pyjamas or nightie, to stop the child sleeping on his or her back. These may not be safe in small children. If the snoring is causing family disruption, consult your doctor. If no one is disturbed by it, ignore it!

USUAL TREATMENT

If the cause is nasal congestion, decongestants may be prescribed. If the adenoids are particularly enlarged, or linked with deafness, your GP may refer your child to an ENT (ear, nose and throat) surgeon for a full assessment.

Soiling

See also Constipation

This is the passing of faeces into clothing after an age at which you would normally expect a child to have bowel control.

SYMPTOMS

Bowel control is usually accomplished by the age of three or four years. However, soiling is not uncommon and, interestingly, more than half the children with this problem also wet the bed. The most common cause is constipation. This occurs because a large, hard motion blocks the bowel and small amounts of softer motion ooze around the side of this and leak out. The problem can be more likely to happen if a child is under stress, but this is not always the case. Children who soil are frequently, and understandably, embarrassed by this and tend to hide their dirty clothes. Another type of soiling is encopresis; in this case, the child deliberately passes motions in inappropriate places.

ACTION

If your child does start to soil, consult your doctor. The doctor will examine your child's abdomen to see whether constipation is the source of the problem, and can offer general advice on how you can best help your child.

USUAL TREATMENT

Both constipation and encopresis are treated with laxatives. Encopresis is also treated by referral for assessment by a child psychologist. The long-term outlook in solving soiling problems is almost always excellent.

Sore Throat

Pain in the throat, which may or may not be linked with other problems such as a cold or earache. One cause of a recurrent sore throat is tonsillitis, when the tonsils (fleshy swellings at the back of the throat that form part of the lymphatic system) become inflamed.

SYMPTOMS

Sore throats are very common. They can occur at every age, and children who are old enough will simply tell you that the throat is sore. Your child may have difficulty in swallowing and have enlarged cervical glands, which are the lymph nodes in the front of the neck. They prevent infection from spreading and swell up when they are doing their job. Some children also get tummy ache at the same time, which is caused by a condition called mesenteric adenitis when the glands in the abdomen swell. In a few cases the pain from this can be quite severe, and it is frequently mistaken for appendicitis.

Most sore throats are mild, and your child may not seem particularly unwell. A sore throat may be part of an ordinary cold, and your doctor may describe it as an 'upper respiratory infection'.

Babies with sore throats often simply seem unwell, or may have a temperature. They may be off their food and they may be reluctant to swallow, but the symptoms will not be specific.

TONSILLITIS
In tonsillitis, the sore throat is likely to be much more severe. The tonsils themselves will be swollen and red and may be covered with white spots of pus. Also, your child may have unpleasant-smelling breath, a high temperature, no appetite and will seem generally under the weather.

Sore Throat

ACTION

You should consult a doctor about a sore throat if:

- The sore throat shows no sign of improvement after four days

- Your child has a headache or is particularly unwell

- Your child develops earache

- Your child comes out in a rash

- You can't keep your child's temperature down

- You are particularly worried about your child's condition

If your child is feverish, you should cool him or her down by removing some clothes and, if necessary, by bathing in tepid water. Offer plenty of drinks, but don't worry if your child doesn't want to eat – a day or two without food will do no harm. If your child is hungry but has difficulty swallowing solid food, give ice cream or liquidized food. Giving paracetamol will help to keep the temperature down, and will soothe the soreness. For most cases of sore throat, this should be all that is required. However, if the symptoms do not settle after four days or so, or if there are other symptoms such as those mentioned above, you should consult your doctor.

USUAL TREATMENT

Approximately 7 out of 10 cases of tonsillitis and sore throats are caused by viruses, for which there is no effective treatment other than painkillers. If the infection is caused by bacteria, on the other hand, then antibiotics may be helpful. But the doctor cannot tell with certainty which sore throats are viral and which are bacterial. Medical opinion on how to treat young children varies widely. Some doctors give antibiotics routinely to a child on the grounds that they might help and probably won't do any harm. Other doctors are more concerned that overuse of antibiotics may result in bacteria becoming more resistant, which could lead to more severe infections for children in the future. Some doctors prefer not to prescribe antibiotics at all, because they feel that they are

Sore Throat

not necessary. The usual approach is a compromise. Your doctor may reserve antibiotics for throat infections that have lasted four or five days with no sign of improvement. He or she may take other factors into account, too. For example, if your child has a part in the school play, or if you are going on holiday tomorrow, he might decide to prescribe antibiotics.

TONSILLITIS

Parents whose children have repeated episodes of tonsillitis often ask if the tonsils can be removed. While tonsillectomy was very common years ago, nowadays we know that the great majority of children grow out of repeated sore throats by the time they are around six, and that in most people the tonsils shrink away to next to nothing. For this reason doctors today are much more selective about whether to recommend a tonsillectomy. There is little point in putting your child through unnecessary surgery, and no operation should be considered lightly.

However, if your child has suffered four or five attacks of tonsillitis a year over the last 18 months, your GP may decide that the tonsils should be removed. Normally, ENT (ear, nose and throat) surgeons prefer to wait until a child is at least four years old before carrying out a tonsillectomy. This is because a younger child will often refuse to swallow solid food after the operation, and it is important for him or her to get back to swallowing as soon as possible, since eating solid food helps to keep the wound clean and prevent infection.

Speech Problems

See also Cleft Lip and Palate ● Deafness

Children vary greatly in the speed with which they learn to talk, but if it becomes apparent that your child is not speaking as well or as distinctly as others of the same age, this might be a sign that there is a speech problem. This particularly applies over the age of three years.

WHAT TO WATCH FOR

TYPICAL STAGES IN LEARNING TO SPEAK ARE AS FOLLOWS:
3 months: child begins to babble
9 months: child begins to copy words, but usually does not understand them
12–18 months: two-word phrases start, such as 'That hot!'
2–3 years: by the age of 3 years, the average length of a sentence is four words. Most sounds will have developed, though the child may still lisp.

OVER THE AGE OF THREE YEARS COMMON SPEECH PROBLEMS CAN INCLUDE ANY OF THE FOLLOWING:
● Lisping: very common when a child is learning to talk. The child with a lisp tends to pronounce 's' as 'th', or 'th' for 'f'. Temporary lisping can occur when a child has lost

his or her front teeth and will soon remedy itself. It can also be linked with a cleft palate.

● Stammering and stuttering: as children first learn to speak they often go through a phase of stuttering, probably because they want to speak more quickly than they are able to. However, if your child persists with a stutter, never ever be cross about it, make fun of it or imitate it as this can make the child embarrassed which will exacerbate the problem. Speech and language therapists can have real success treating this problem.

● Mispronunciation of words: again, this is very common in the initial stages of learning to talk and usually improves with time. However, if a child

Speech Problems

cannot hear how words are pronounced, he or she will have no way of knowing how to say them. Deafness, caused by conditions such as glue ear, can be a major factor in many types of speech problem.

ACTION

Talk to your child as much as you can from birth so that your child can develop a fascination for language. Children learn to talk by listening to others. If a child is understimulated he will not be as advanced as other children of the same age when it comes to talking. Children need to be told stories, sung to and talked to all the time – even if they are too young to appear to understand. If you are concerned about your child's speech, first of all consult your GP who will examine your child, paying particular attention to the ears and checking for nasal congestion or enlarged adenoids, both of which may affect a child's hearing.

USUAL TREATMENT

Your doctor may refer your child for a hearing assessment, followed by an appointment with an ENT (ear, nose and throat) specialist if hearing problems seem to be the cause. If this is not the case, your GP will refer your child to a speech and language therapist for further assessment. It may be that no further treatment is required and your child simply has a slight delay in speaking and will catch up in time.

If the cause of the problem is enlarged adenoids or even glue ear, then surgery to remedy these problems will be the most appropriate treatment, although the initial treatment of glue ear is usually antibiotics.

Spina Bifida

A congenital defect in which part of one or more vertebrae fails to develop completely, leaving a gap, so that in extreme cases the nerves of the spinal cord are exposed. There are three main types of spina bifida. Spina bifida occulta: this is the most common, and the least serious form. It often causes no symptoms or problems. Myelocoele: this is the most severe form, and a child with this will be severely handicapped from birth. Meningocoele: the covering of the spinal cord is exposed, but the nerve tissue is intact and usually undamaged.

SYMPTOMS

Symptoms depend on severity:

- Swelling of the spine
- Exposure of part of the spinal cord
- Dimple or brown hairy mole at the base of the spine
- Paralysis below the waist
- Incontinence
- Large head (hydrocephalus)

ACTION

Severe spina bifida will be apparent from birth. Surgery can be carried out to correct the defect but this will not restore the function of the spinal cord. However, less severe cases may just need surgical repair followed by physiotherapy.

USUAL TREATMENT

Physiotherapy and surgery might be required. Make sure you get adequate information about your child's problem, and consider genetic counselling before deciding to have another child. Folic acid supplements during early pregnancy reduce the risk of the disorder.

Sprains

See also Fractures

Sprains are caused by sudden stretching or slight tearing of the ligaments that hold together the bones in and around a joint; for example, when a child trips, twisting the ankle by going over on the outside of the foot and placing the whole body weight on the ankle, thus stretching or tearing the ligament.

SYMPTOMS

The main symptom of spraining is swelling of the joint. Moving the joint is likely to be painful.

ACTION

If you think that your child has suffered a sprain, seek medical help. Sprains can be made more comfortable if you remember the word RICE. This stands for:

- Rest: avoid moving the joint.
- Ice: apply an ice pack to reduce swelling and pain.
- Compression: apply a firm bandage to support and ease the joint and reduce bruising.
- Elevation: raise the affected limb; for example, rest a twisted ankle on a foot stool, to reduce swelling.

USUAL TREATMENT

Unless there is a wound or the limb is misshapen, the 'RICE' technique can make a sprain much more comfortable while you are waiting to see a doctor. Severe spraining will be treated by firm strapping, though an x-ray may be taken if your doctor suspects the possibility of a fracture.

Squint

Both eyes should look in exactly the same direction and be perfectly parallel. Squint is the term used when the eyes are looking in different directions. There are several causes, such as muscle imbalance or long-sightedness.

WHAT TO WATCH FOR

It is not uncommon for new babies to have an occasional squint. At about three months the eyes should become perfectly aligned. If squinting persists before or after this, it needs assessing and treating. Normally the brain combines the information received from the two eyes in a single image. If the eyes are not perfectly in synch with each other, the brain cannot do this and the child will see double. The brain copes with this double image by suppressing the weaker one altogether. A squint that goes untreated will cause loss of vision in one of the eyes.

ACTION

It is essential that all children with a squint are assessed by a doctor. Quite a lot of apparent squints are an optical illusion caused by a broad bridge of the nose but, even so, do not hesitate to consult your GP.

USUAL TREATMENT

If your doctor confirms the presence of a squint, he or she will refer your child for a full assessment by a hospital orthoptic or ophthalmology department. Treatment will then depend on the cause but could include putting a patch over one eye, the prescribing of glasses if a visual problem such as long-sightedness is the cause, or, more rarely, surgery.

Sudden Infant Death Syndrome

The sudden, unexplained death of an apparently normal baby. This most commonly occurs between two and four months and is extremely rare over the age of seven months.

EVERY PARENT'S NIGHTMARE

There cannot be a parent who does not have nightmares about this dreadful condition, in which an apparently healthy baby dies suddenly, usually during the night, and for no discernible reason. Although there has been a dramatic reduction in deaths over the last 5–10 years, with a 60 per cent reduction in the UK since 1991, there are still about 10 deaths every week nationally. Do try to remember that the chance of it actually happening to your baby is still remote and very low.

CAUSES AND RISKS

In the past the condition was known as cot death, which somehow implied that cots were the cause, or that a cot was the only place that this might happen. In fact, sudden infant death can occur at any time, and the term Sudden Infant Death Syndrome, or SIDS, is a technical term that stresses the fact that a cause of death was not discovered. It is likely that there may be many different causes.

Although almost everything from chemical gases, mattresses and vaccinations has been claimed as the cause of SIDS, none of these environmental factors has any proven scientific validity. However, there are three situations which do increase the risk. These are:

- Smoking: babies whose parents smoke either during the pregnancy or afterwards, or particularly both, are at significantly higher risk of cot death.

- Overheating: if a baby becomes too hot in the cot or bed, this also increases the risk.

- Position: lying the baby face down also increases the risk.

Sudden Infant Death Syndrome

PREVENTION

Avoiding the known risk factors can certainly reduce your baby's risk of SIDS. The advice is simple:

- Avoid smoking.

- Do not allow your baby to become overheated. Make up the cot so that your baby's feet are almost touching the foot end, with the bedclothes arranged so that they only cover half of the cot. This means that the baby cannot snuggle down under the bedclothes and become overheated.

- Put your baby to sleep on his or her back (remember the slogan 'back to sleep').

- Breast-feed your baby if at all possible. There is evidence that breast-feeding helps to protect against infections, and infections may be implicated in SIDS in some cases.

IF IT HAPPENED TO YOUR BABY...

The feeling of grief, mixed with tremendous guilt, can be completely overwhelming. Unkind comments that link the condition to smothering, or even the feeling that it must be possible to prevent SIDS if only they had tried hard enough, make parents feel devastatingly guilty and inadequate. In fact, it is vital to realize that the preventive advice is not guaranteed to be effective. Sadly there are SIDS parents who followed this advice and still lost their child.

Because the overall cause is unknown, no parent should ever blame themselves for not having done enough to prevent their baby's death. We know that death, when it occurs, appears to take place within seconds and typically happens during sleep so the baby does not suffer. The family suffers dreadfully, however. Trying to understand better what has happened is very important. Both counselling and talking to other parents in the same situation will be extremely helpful in coping with your feelings.

Sunburn and Sun Protection

Inflammation and blistering of the skin can be caused by excessive exposure to sunshine. There are few sights that are sadder than a badly burned baby or small child on a supposedly happy family holiday. Sunburn is entirely preventable and the responsibility of parents.

SYMPTOMS

The main symptoms are pain and redness, itching and peeling skin, and, if severe, blistering. People often trivialize sunburn, but it is a genuine burn and precautions should be taken to prevent it.

ACTION

Prevention is everything. Sunburn is very painful and can increase the likelihood of later development of skin cancer. You aren't being a killjoy by keeping your child in a T-shirt and, whenever possible, a sun hat. In addition, always use plenty of high-factor, total-block sunscreen, and only slowly allow increased sun exposure, ideally to no more than 30 minutes in a session. Children with fair complexions are particularly at risk and should always avoid direct contact with the sun if at all possible. Make sure that there is always accessible shade, and remember that children can get burnt in water. See a doctor if blistering occurs or if there is severe pain, dizziness or fever.

USUAL TREATMENT

Prevention is by far the best plan, but if your child does become sunburnt, cool water and calamine lotion can be very soothing. Keep your child out of the sun for 48 hours. In the case of severe burns your doctor may advise hydrocortisone cream. Do not use creams that contain local anaesthetic as these can slow healing.

Swollen Glands

See also Cancer ● Sore Throat ● Tonsillitis

Lymph glands are spread around the body and act as part of the body's defence against infection. If there is an infection in the body, the lymph glands frequently swell.

SYMPTOMS

If your child has an infection, the lymph glands in the neck, armpits and groin may swell. For instance, if your child has a throat infection, the glands in the neck will swell slightly to prevent the infection spreading elsewhere, such as the lungs. Glands might stay swollen for a couple of weeks after an infection, but should not be tender after a few days.

ACTION

If a swelling appears red and painful as well as being swollen, then seek your doctor's advice today. In addition, if any swollen gland persists for about two weeks, then ask your doctor to check it. Although it is relatively uncommon, small children do sometimes get glandular fever. It can only be diagnosed by a blood test. Very rarely, persistent swollen glands might be linked with leukaemia.

USUAL TREATMENT

An infected gland which is red and warm might need antibiotics, but most infections causing simple swelling do not.

Teething

The process of teeth coming through in babies and small children can cause pain and tenderness in the gums.

WHAT TO WATCH FOR

Teeth begin to develop well before they appear in the mouth. The initial stages of development start before birth, and the first teeth to appear are the incisors, the teeth at the very front of the mouth. Typically the 20 primary teeth will have appeared by the age of two-and-a-half years. Some babies are born with one or more teeth already showing. As the tooth is coming through the gum, the gum becomes red and inflamed and sometimes a blister may cover the tooth as it first pokes through the surface. There is no evidence whatsoever that problems such as diarrhoea, rashes or coughs are associated with teething – these just happen to be common at about the same age. The only things that teething causes are dribbling, discomfort, irritability – and teeth.

ACTION

Some babies find that chewing on a hard, smooth object, such as a teething ring or scrubbed carrot can help. However, never leave your baby alone with any of these in case he or she chokes. Rusks are acceptable if they are sugar-free.

USUAL TREATMENT

You are unlikely to need to consult a doctor about teething. However, paracetamol liquid and cuddles for comfort may be helpful. For babies over four months you might try a teething gel. Make sure that any gel you use is sugar-free and does not contain aspirin.

Terrible Twos

See also Sibling Rivalry

A phase of temper tantrums and total lack of co-operation, which usually happens at around the age of two.

WHAT TO WATCH FOR

At around the age of two your child is beginning to assert him- or herself for the first time. Two-year-olds have every right to think that the world revolves around them. When things begin to change, as they must, they don't like it. They react with angry and unco-operative behaviour, often crying and kicking.

ACTION

It is tempting to give way to any outburst of temper, particularly if it happens in the middle of a crowded supermarket. However, this teaches your child that tantrums pay. Instead, make it clear that your child will be ignored until he or she calms down. Two-year-olds hate being ignored and they will quickly learn that the best way to get your attention again is to quieten down. The most effective way of teaching them this is by using the 'time out' technique: very calmly pick up your child and put him or her in another room until good behaviour is restored.

USUAL TREATMENT

In general, temper tantrums usually fade by the time the child reaches his or her fourth birthday. If you find that the 'time out' technique, or ignoring your child, or even offering a distraction whenever a tantrum seems imminent, does not work, then talk to your health visitor or your GP.

Testicle – undescended

Before or shortly after birth the testicles normally move down from inside the abdomen to the scrotum, the sac of skin that holds the testicles outside the body. If one testicle fails to appear, then this is described as an 'undescended testicle'.

WHAT TO WATCH FOR

If you want to check whether your child's testicles are in the scrotum, then a warm bath is the ideal opportunity. Many boys also have retractile testicles that appear and disappear from the scrotum like a yo-yo. This is because the testicles are attached to sensitive muscles, which pull the testicles up if they are exposed to cold or if the child is embarrassed at being exposed. If a testicle appears to be undescended but can sometimes be found in the scrotum, then there is rarely any cause for concern. If it *can* be there, it will be there when it matters.

ACTION

In most cases, testicles that are undescended at birth will have dropped down by the age of seven months. If you are still concerned after this age or if one of your son's testicles never appears in the scrotum, then you should talk to your doctor.

USUAL TREATMENT

A permanently undescended testicle can become damaged and fertility problems might occur in later life, so a simple operation should be carried out in the first few years to lower the testicle into its normal position. However, most boys who appear to have undescended testicles in fact turn out just to have retractile testicles and no treatment is needed at all.

Threadworms

These tiny worms infest the intestines and bowel. They are so named because they look like pieces of cotton thread. They are incredibly common, and are neither harmful nor a sign of any negligence on your part.

SYMPTOMS

The chief symptom of threadworms is anal itching, and possible itching of the vagina in girls. You may see the worms on your child's buttocks or in motions. Threadworms do not cause any other illness or weight loss. They live in the bowel, and at night the females emerge through the anus to lay their eggs on the skin around the anus. This leads to itching, scratching and possibly disturbed sleep. The child will almost certainly then get the threadworm eggs on his or her finger, and then put the fingers in the mouth so swallowing more eggs and worsening the condition. The problem is extremely infectious and doctors usually treat the whole family.

ACTION

If you are sure of the diagnosis, you can get a preparation to treat the worms from your doctor or pharmacist. If you are unsure of the cause of anal itching, see your doctor.

USUAL TREATMENT

Medication taken as a single dose is usually repeated a couple of weeks later. Check with your doctor if any child needing treatment is aged under one year. Make sure that bedding and pyjamas are washed to clear away any remaining eggs. Scrupulous hygiene, trimming of fingernails and treating the whole family will lead to rapid recovery.

Tics and Twitches

A tic is a quick, sudden movement or the making of a sound. The movements or sounds appear to be deliberate and usually occur in the same part of the child's face or body. Some tics and twitches can be controlled, others cannot.

SYMPTOMS

Tics and twitches are very common, especially around the age that a child starts school. The most common examples are blinking, sniffing, flicking of the head, clearing the throat with a small cough or grunting. The child can often repeat the movements deliberately on request, and can stop them if he or she really thinks about it. Tics are more likely to occur when the child is inactive and will frequently disappear when he or she is concentrating. Other persistent tics may be involuntary (chronic tic disorder). Vocal tics such as hooting, yelping or swearing are possible signs of the very rare neurological condition called Gilles de la Tourette's syndrome.

ACTION

Tics and twitches are often made much worse by anxiety or stress, so the less attention that parents pay to them, the better. Most tics and twitches will usually clear up without any treatment, and reassurance is the most important initial step.

USUAL TREATMENT

Most tics and twitches disappear eventually but, if they seem to get worse, consult your doctor who may refer your child for behavioural therapy or further assessment. Gilles de la Tourette's syndrome and other similar rare cases may require medication and behavioural therapy.

Toilet Training

See also Bedwetting ● Urinary Tract Infections

Most children are fully toilet-trained by the time they are three or four years old, with daytime success occurring about six months before night-time control. There is nothing you can do to speed this process up, but criticism can certainly slow things down. Up to 15 per cent, mostly boys, will continue to be wet at night on a regular basis up to the age of five years or older.

WHAT TO WATCH FOR

Start to introduce the potty and encourage your child to sit on it when he or she begins to show signs of being aware of having a full bladder or being about to pass a motion.

TIPS FOR SUCCESS

The best ways to encourage toilet training are:

● Praise your child for trying, and ignore mistakes.

● Make toilet training fun: applause, encouragement and even a potty with a favourite cartoon character will make the experience less stressful.

● When your child is able to control urination and bowel movements for several hours, suggest that he or she use the potty or a seat on the toilet.

● If your child has been dry for three or four nights, try leaving the nappy off but be prepared for accidents by using a plastic sheet on the mattress.

● If your child starts wetting again when you try this, revert to putting a nappy on every night for another couple of weeks, then try again.

Toothache

Pain in a tooth or gum is most typically caused by tooth decay, which should be nearly completely preventable.

SYMPTOMS

Pain from toothache can be constant and throbbing, or may just give twinges of pain that occur with certain stimuli, such as very cold drinks or ice. The gum near the tooth may be swollen and tender. If putting pressure on a tooth or tapping it triggers pain, there is almost certainly tooth decay present.

ACTION

The diagnosis of toothache is usually very straightforward, and the immediate treatment is to give paracetamol. Warmth (such as from a hot water bottle wrapped in a towel) or even an icepack on the cheek can also help to ease the pain. Contact your dentist to have the tooth or teeth examined and ask for an emergency appointment. If you cannot contact your usual dentist and the pain is very bad, your local hospital should have a list of emergency dentists, as should your local GP out-of-hours service.

USUAL TREATMENT

The dentist will assess the cause of the toothache and treat any tooth decay as required, perhaps with a filling or antibiotics if there is an infection. Discuss with your dentist whether your child should be using a fluoride toothpaste or taking fluoride supplements. In the long term it is very important to encourage your child to take really good care of his or her teeth by regular brushing and regular check-ups with your dentist.

Travel Sickness

This occurs because the balance mechanism in the ear is sensitive to repeated movements, such as those made by a car or boat. Small babies rarely seem to suffer, but motion sickness is possible before the age of six months.

SYMPTOMS

The main symptoms are nausea and dizziness, sometimes leading to vomiting. Some children go very pale.

ACTION

- Make sure that your child can see out of the front window, using a booster seat if necessary. Everything seems to be moving faster out of the side, making the problem worse.

- Try to ensure that he or she does not spend the journey looking down at toys or books.

- Avoid large meals or drinks before the journey. Small, dry snacks, such as biscuits or crackers, help, as do sweets which can be sucked.

- Sit over a coach's centre of gravity to keep lateral and vertical movements to a minimum.

- Small children are less likely to be sick if they have something to rest their feet on, rather than leaving them dangling.

USUAL TREATMENT

If all else fails, talk to your doctor or pharmacist about travel sickness medication. If this doesn't work, an empty ice-cream container makes the perfect bowl in case sickness occurs – cheap, disposable and with an air-tight lid!

Tuberculosis

Tuberculosis, or TB, is a serious infectious disease, and can take many different forms. The most common form of TB is pulmonary tuberculosis, which affects the lungs, and is spread from an infected person who coughs or sneezes bacteria in airborne droplets.

SYMPTOMS

Symptoms include fever, loss of appetite, cough, pallor, sweating and lack of energy, all of which may persist for weeks or months.

ACTION

A mass screening and immunization programme mainly aimed at teenagers has helped reduce the incidence of TB spreading to children. However, if you have been in contact with anyone with TB, or have travelled to an area where TB is a major problem, and your child develops any suspicious symptoms, then consult your doctor right away so that screening and diagnostic tests can be performed right away.

USUAL TREATMENT

If your child is diagnosed as having TB, which will often be done with a chest x-ray, he or she will be referred to a specialist for treatment. Modern anti-tuberculous drugs are extremely effective, but this does not in any way reduce the need for careful screening to prevent outbreaks occurring.

Tummy Ache

See also Appendicitis ● Colic ● Constipation
● Diarrhoea ● Gastroenteritis ● Intussusception
● Urinary Tract Infections

Abdominal pain in children can be a one-off episode (known as 'acute' pain) or it may be recurrent (known as 'chronic' pain).

SYMPTOMS

Tummy ache must be one of the most common complaints in childhood and it usually fades away harmlessly. Acute abdominal pain is frequently associated with diarrhoea and sickness, and there are any number of possible causes from constipation to appendicitis. The most common cause of recurrent abdominal pain is a curious condition known as the 'periodic syndrome'. The cause is uncertain, but the condition affects up to 15 per cent of school-aged children. The pain is usually worse in the day but does not disturb sleep at night. It can continue on and off for months. Some children seem to be either more sensitive to the normal contractions of the gut ('peristalsis') or have stronger than average contractions. The pain of periodic syndrome is not caused by constipation, although constipation can sometimes result from the condition.

ACTION

All children with recurrent abdominal pain should be assessed by a doctor, even though frequently all tests are negative. In particular, every child with recurrent abdominal pain should have his or her urine examined to make sure that there is no sign of infection. If a pain occurs only on Monday mornings before school, for instance, then it is highly unlikely that there is any physical cause, but a check-up by

Tummy Ache

the doctor will still help you in managing the problem.

There are certain times when you should call a doctor immediately if your child is experiencing acute abdominal pain. These are:

- If the pain is severe and does not ease up

- If the pain is constant for more than a couple of hours

- If pain that was crampy becomes constant

- If your child continues to retch even after there is nothing left to bring up

- If your child seems to be very ill

- If it hurts when you press on your child's abdomen

- If your child's abdomen is swollen

- If there has been a recent injury of any sort to the abdomen

- If your child's abdomen feels rock-hard

- If a boy has any pain in the testicles

- If there is blood in your child's motions or vomit

USUAL TREATMENT

The treatment of acute abdominal pain depends very much on its cause. When any physical cause has been ruled out, recurrent tummy ache can be difficult to deal with. It is sometimes helpful to consider this type of tummy ache as the child's equivalent of an adult headache: however carefully a doctor examined the adult during such a pain, he would find no physical abnormality even though the pain is very real. The same goes for many tummy aches in children. Paracetamol can be very helpful, as can a hot water bottle and a lot of sympathy.

Bear in mind the possibility of a food allergy or intolerance as a cause of the symptoms. Keep a food diary to see if there is any particular food that triggers the symptoms. In all cases, if the symptoms change, go back to your doctor.

Turner's Syndrome

A chromosomal abnormality present from birth that affects only girls (1 in every 3000), so it is not common, but neither is it exceptionally rare. Children normally have 46 chromosomes, but typically in Turner's syndrome one chromosome is missing.

SYMPTOMS

A girl with Turner's syndrome is short, with webbing of the skin of the neck, absent or very retarded development of secondary sexual characteristics, abnormalities of the eyes and the bones, and frequently a degree of mental retardation. There may be a condition known as coarctation of the aorta, which is a narrowing of the main artery from the heart, causing headache and poor circulation.

ACTION

If the condition is a possibility, then your child will be referred for chromosomal analysis and full assessment by a consultant paediatrician.

USUAL TREATMENT

There is no treatment for the underlying chromosomal abnormality, but treatment in adolescence with oestrogens can help the development of secondary sexual characteristics, such as breast development and menstruation. Sadly, there is no possibility of such girls ever becoming pregnant. The coarctation of the aorta is corrected with surgery at an early age.

If this condition is diagnosed you will find it very helpful to find out as much as possible about the syndrome. The self-help organizations and your doctor will be able to advise on special educational or medical needs if these are required.

Umbilical Cord Problems

See also Lumps

A protruding tummy button, or umbilical hernia, is a common parental concern. The umbilicus (the medical term for tummy button or navel) is the remains of the umbilical cord that connects the baby to the placenta before birth. Its size can depend on a number of factors, including the way in which it was cut and tied after birth.

SYMPTOMS

Babies often have a small hernia, or weakness of the underlying muscle, so that the lump bulges. This does not usually cause problems. The only time to be concerned is when it becomes strangulated, and the lump rock hard and impossible to push back in. The baby would be unwell and vomiting repeatedly. However, this is extremely rare.

ACTION

The vast majority of newborn umbilical hernias are harmless and disappear by themselves. A very small number persist without getting smaller. If you are concerned that your baby has a strangulated hernia, contact your doctor without delay.

USUAL TREATMENT

If an umbilical hernia persists, then it can be corrected surgically.

n, or immunization, programme has been ...rotect children, and the community, against a ...tially serious and dangerous illnesses.

...ES

...worries about their child having vaccinations. ...t having the injection actually is the bigger risk – ...your child could contract one of the diseases the ...are designed to prevent.

...MUNIZATION WORKS

...born with some natural immunity from their ...d this is also topped up through breastfeeding. ...the baby's own immune system begins to develop. ...ny dose of the virus by vaccination will stimulate the ...y to produce antibodies against that virus. If the child ...osed to that virus, the antibodies will be there, ready ...f infection.

...HOULD NOT BE IMMUNIZED?

...ld always let the doctor, health visitor or nurse know if ...d:

...high fever

...had a bad reaction to a previous immunization ...ugh this may not mean that other injections cannot be ...n)

...had, or is having, cancer treatment, or is on any ...dicine which affects the immune system, including ...munosuppressant therapy or high-dose steroids

...s any form of bleeding disorder

Urinary Tract Infections

See also Tummy Ache

A urinary tract infection (often abbreviated to UTI) refers to an infection in the urine, bladder, urethra (the tube through which urine leaves the body), ureters (the tubes that lead from the kidney to the bladder) or kidneys. Bacteria almost always get into the bladder from the bowel, and because the urethra is so much shorter in girls than boys and nearer to the anus, they are affected more than boys. Approximately 1 in 20 girls will have a UTI before they reach puberty. If the infection only affects the bladder, this is called cystitis. If the infection gets up the ureters to one or both kidneys, pyelonephritis is diagnosed.

SYMPTOMS

The main symptoms of a urinary tract infection may be any of the following:

- Frequency (passing urine more frequently than normal)
- Pain on passing urine
- Unpleasant-smelling urine
- Blood in the urine
- Back pain
- Tummy ache, which can be very vague and nondescript
- Fever
- Bedwetting

- A baby who is vaguely unwell, possibly off his or her food, or vomiting, or who has diarrhoea

CONTACT YOUR DOCTOR URGENTLY IF:
- Your child's temperature is over 38.3°C/102°F
- If your child is complaining of abdominal pain
- If there is blood in your child's urine, or
- If your child seems particularly unwell

Urinary Tract Infections

ACTION

Every small child who might have a urinary infection must be seen by a doctor. There should be no exceptions. The diagnosis is not always easy to make just from the symptoms described above. The urine has to be examined to confirm the presence or absence of infection. If an infection is present, your child will be investigated to make sure there is no abnormality of the urinary tract, such as a problem with the valve at the bottom of the ureter. It is vitally important to know that there is no risk of recurrent infections, or of any long-term damage to the kidneys. You should always consult a doctor if there is any possibility of urine infection in your child, taking a specimen of your child's urine with you when you see the doctor. Your GP may test the specimen at the surgery and is also likely to send it to a laboratory, where it will be examined. Any bacteria found will be cultured to determine which antibiotics will be effective.

USUAL TREATMENT

If you suspect a urinary tract infection, as well as consulting a doctor you should strongly encourage your child to drink as much as possible. This helps to flush the kidneys and bladder out. Antibiotics are also essential for the treatment of proven infections. The potential for long-term kidney damage in urinary tract infections is very real and can cause your child major problems for the rest of his or her life if left untreated.

If an infection is confirmed, children aged under five will always have this investigated further, usually using an ultrasound scan to look at the kidneys, ureters and bladder (known as a KUB scan). This scan can show exactly what the problem might be. Incidentally, infections that occur after the age of six years are very unlikely indeed to lead to kidney damage, and so investigation is much less important.

See also Allergy ● Rashes

A very itchy, raised rash, somet
children will have an attack at s
always triggered by an allergy or
triggers are foods (especially she
medication, insect bites, and expo

SYMPTOMS

The raised rash (see pages 160–2, and illustration between pages 128 and 129) itches dreadfully and individual patches tend to come and go. A single lesion never lasts more than 12 hours. Although most urticaria only

las
hav
peri
part
urtic
exerci
tempe

ACTION

If the rash is accompanied by difficulty in breathing, or if the tongue or inside of the mouth is affected, seek medical help

immedia
not an en
antihistar

USUAL TREATMENT

Antihistamines such as Piriton (chlorpheniramin
treatment. Calamine can help soothe the itching.
what triggered the urticaria so that future attacks

Vaccina

The vaccinatio
developed to p
range of poten

ANXIETI

Every parent
However, no
the risk that
vaccinations

HOW IM

Babies are b
mother, an
Eventually
Giving a ti
baby's bo
is later exp
to fight o

WHO S

You shou
your chi

● Has
● Has
  (tho
  give
● Has
  me
  im
● Ha

- Has had a severe allergic reaction to eggs
- Has had convulsions in the past
- Has HIV or Aids

WILL THERE BE SIDE-EFFECTS?

Most children will not be affected at all apart from a small red and swollen area at the injection site. Some children develop a temperature. Talk to your doctor or nurse about giving a dose of paracetamol if this happens. Very rarely an allergic reaction can occur. If you are at all worried about your child after a vaccination, contact your doctor at once.

WHAT ABOUT MMR?

Parents tend to be very worried about the MMR (measles, mumps and rubella) vaccine. However, around the world 1–2 million children die every year from measles, and even in the UK previously healthy children can die from this illness. If your child is not immunized, he or she will be relying on other people to have their children immunized, and the more children who are not immunized the greater the risks of outbreaks. Scares about the vaccine have mainly been linked to the risk of encephalitis, or inflammation of the brain. Although this has occasionally been reported, the risk of vaccinated children developing encephalitis is no higher than the risk for unvaccinated children. The risk of any child developing encephalitis if they have measles is 1 in 5000, and a third of these will be left with permanent brain damage. Not having the vaccine is by far the greater risk.

Vaginal Discharge

See also Foreign Bodies

The internal skin of the vagina is much more sensitive in small girls than it is after puberty, and so many irritants can lead to a vaginal discharge and possibly itching. Irritants include bubble bath, fabric conditioners, tight clothing and foreign bodies in the vagina. Rolled-up toilet paper, peanuts, crayons and almost anything may be inserted, and they can act as the focus for infection and result in a vaginal discharge.

SYMPTOMS

If your daughter is rubbing or scratching the vaginal area and/or has a persistent vaginal discharge that is strongly smelling, dark in colour or bloody, see your doctor who will probably take a swab to find out what bacteria are causing the problem.

ACTION

If the foreign body is half protruding and has no sharp edges, you may be able to get it out. However, if in doubt don't try: you may make matters worse. Consult a doctor, who will have suitable instruments. If this happens again, seek advice. Repeated insertion of a foreign body might be a sign of emotional disturbance, or even of sexual abuse.

USUAL TREATMENT

Depending on the results of any swabs, antibiotic medicine or appropriate creams may be prescribed. Encourage good hygiene: scratching the bottom and vulval area with dirty fingers is a common childhood activity, but is not a good idea.

Urinary Tract Infections

See also Tummy Ache

A urinary tract infection (often abbreviated to UTI) refers to an infection in the urine, bladder, urethra (the tube through which urine leaves the body), ureters (the tubes that lead from the kidney to the bladder) or kidneys. Bacteria almost always get into the bladder from the bowel, and because the urethra is so much shorter in girls than boys and nearer to the anus, they are affected more than boys. Approximately 1 in 20 girls will have a UTI before they reach puberty. If the infection only affects the bladder, this is called cystitis. If the infection gets up the ureters to one or both kidneys, pyelonephritis is diagnosed.

SYMPTOMS

The main symptoms of a urinary tract infection may be any of the following:

- Frequency (passing urine more frequently than normal)

- Pain on passing urine

- Unpleasant-smelling urine

- Blood in the urine

- Back pain

- Tummy ache, which can be very vague and nondescript

- Fever

- Bedwetting

- A baby who is vaguely unwell, possibly off his or her food, or vomiting, or who has diarrhoea

CONTACT YOUR DOCTOR URGENTLY IF:
- Your child's temperature is over 38.3°C/102°F

- If your child is complaining of abdominal pain

- If there is blood in your child's urine, or

- If your child seems particularly unwell

Urinary Tract Infections

ACTION

Every small child who might have a urinary infection must be seen by a doctor. There should be no exceptions. The diagnosis is not always easy to make just from the symptoms described above. The urine has to be examined to confirm the presence or absence of infection. If an infection is present, your child will be investigated to make sure there is no abnormality of the urinary tract, such as a problem with the valve at the bottom of the ureter. It is vitally important to know that there is no risk of recurrent infections, or of any long-term damage to the kidneys. You should always consult a doctor if there is any possibility of urine infection in your child, taking a specimen of your child's urine with you when you see the doctor. Your GP may test the specimen at the surgery and is also likely to send it to a laboratory, where it will be examined. Any bacteria found will be cultured to determine which antibiotics will be effective.

USUAL TREATMENT

If you suspect a urinary tract infection, as well as consulting a doctor you should strongly encourage your child to drink as much as possible. This helps to flush the kidneys and bladder out. Antibiotics are also essential for the treatment of proven infections. The potential for long-term kidney damage in urinary tract infections is very real and can cause your child major problems for the rest of his or her life if left untreated.

If an infection is confirmed, children aged under five will always have this investigated further, usually using an ultrasound scan to look at the kidneys, ureters and bladder (known as a KUB scan). This scan can show exactly what the problem might be. Incidentally, infections that occur after the age of six years are very unlikely indeed to lead to kidney damage, and so investigation is much less important.

Urticaria

See also Allergy ● Rashes

A very itchy, raised rash, sometimes known as hives. One in five children will have an attack at some stage and it is almost always triggered by an allergy of some sort. The most common triggers are foods (especially shellfish or strawberries), medication, insect bites, and exposure to certain plants.

SYMPTOMS

The raised rash (see pages 160–2, and illustration between pages 128 and 129) itches dreadfully and individual patches tend to come and go. A single lesion never lasts more than 12 hours. Although most urticaria only lasts a few days, some children have repeated attacks over a period of time. This can occur in particular with the rarer types of urticaria which appear after exercise or an increase in temperature.

ACTION

If the rash is accompanied by difficulty in breathing, or if the tongue or inside of the mouth is affected, seek medical help immediately. If the situation is not an emergency, antihistamines may suffice.

USUAL TREATMENT

Antihistamines such as Piriton (chlorpheniramine) are the chief treatment. Calamine can help soothe the itching. Try to work out what triggered the urticaria so that future attacks can be avoided.

Vaccination

The vaccination, or immunization, programme has been developed to protect children, and the community, against a range of potentially serious and dangerous illnesses.

ANXIETIES

Every parent worries about their child having vaccinations. However, not having the injection actually is the bigger risk – the risk that your child could contract one of the diseases the vaccinations are designed to prevent.

HOW IMMUNIZATION WORKS

Babies are born with some natural immunity from their mother, and this is also topped up through breastfeeding. Eventually the baby's own immune system begins to develop. Giving a tiny dose of the virus by vaccination will stimulate the baby's body to produce antibodies against that virus. If the child is later exposed to that virus, the antibodies will be there, ready to fight off infection.

WHO SHOULD NOT BE IMMUNIZED?

You should always let the doctor, health visitor or nurse know if your child:

- Has a high fever
- Has had a bad reaction to a previous immunization (though this may not mean that other injections cannot be given)
- Has had, or is having, cancer treatment, or is on any medicine which affects the immune system, including immunosuppressant therapy or high-dose steroids
- Has any form of bleeding disorder

Vomiting

See also Dehydration ● Diarrhoea ● Gastroenteritis ● Pyloric Stenosis ● Travel Sickness

Vomiting can occur by itself or with diarrhoea. Sudden onset vomiting is most likely to be linked with some sort of infection, or even more serious conditions such as meningitis.

SYMPTOMS

If the cause is an infection, your child will probably have a raised temperature, and other symptoms which should aid diagnosis.

ACTION

Consult a doctor urgently for:

- Vomiting with any sign of dehydration
- Persistent projectile vomiting
- Vomiting with headache, earache or neck stiffness
- Vomiting with severe abdominal pain
- Blood in the vomit
- Vomiting after a head injury

- If your child's abdomen seems hard, swollen or seems tender to the touch
- Vomiting in a child who appears ill
- Vomiting in a baby for more than six hours
- Vomiting in an older child for more than 12 hours
- If your child vomits even when he or she has taken no food or drink

USUAL TREATMENT

Fluid replacement is essential (see Diarrhoea and Gastroenteritis).

Warts

Warts are harmless thickenings of the outer layer of the skin and are caused by a viral infection. On the soles of the feet they are known as verrucae.

SYMPTOMS

Warts can be found almost anywhere on the body and cause a swelling or lump in the skin. They are usually not painful, but warts on the soles of the feet may become sore simply because the feet are weight-bearing. The most common sites for warts are the feet, the hands and the fingers, especially around the fingernails. They may occur singly, or there may be a cluster of so-called mosaic warts.

ACTION

If warts are painless, you can safely ignore them. Nearly 50 per cent disappear without treatment within 6 to 12 months. Unsightly or painful warts can be treated with over-the-counter or prescribed wart removers in the form of paints, gels or plasters. If these don't work, consult your doctor. Always consult a doctor about warts that are near the anus or the genitals. Never attempt to treat these yourself.

USUAL TREATMENT

If skin treatments have been unsuccessful, then cryosurgery can be used. This technique involves freezing the wart with liquid nitrogen, which can be sprayed or touched onto the wart. This treatment is actually a carefully controlled cold burn, and can be uncomfortable, so most doctors are reluctant to carry it out on very young children.

Wind

See also Colic

Small babies frequently burp loudly after being fed, bringing up any air they may have swallowed while feeding.

SYMPTOMS

Both breast-fed and bottle-fed babies swallow air during feeding, and it is this swallowed air that is produced when you burp your baby. It is *not* gas produced in the stomach.

ACTION

There is no harm in winding your baby, but it is not essential. If a breast-fed baby is swallowing a lot of air, this may be because he or she is not properly latched on to the breast. In bottle-fed babies you may see a lot of air bubbles in the bottle. The only real problem that all this swallowed air can cause is that it makes the baby feel full and bloated, and so may stop feeding before having had enough to eat. This may result in crying for another feed sooner rather than later.

USUAL TREATMENT

If your baby is happy when feeding, do not interrupt the feed to bring his or her wind up. This is completely unnecessary. In addition, if your baby is content after a feed, do not keep patting his back until he burps. If he hasn't swallowed any air, he won't need to bring any up. If you have a windy baby, see if you can adjust the angle you use when feeding to prevent as much air being swallowed.

Useful Organizations

The organizations listed here all provide excellent and valuable help for parents. Most of them are run on tight budgets, so please enclose return postage when contacting them by post.

ASTHMA
The National Asthma Campaign
Providence House
Providence Place
London N1 0NT
Helpline: 0845 7 01 02 03

CANCER
BACUP (British Association of Cancer United Patients)
3 Bath Place,
London EC2
Tel: 0171 613 2121

Leukaemia Society
PO Box 82
Exeter
Devon EX4 8JN
Tel: 01392 464848
Local rate tel: 0345 673203

CEREBRAL PALSY
Scope – for people with cerebral palsy
PO Box 833
Milton Keynes
Bucks MK12 5NY
Tel: 0800 626216

CRYING
Serene (formerly the Cry-Sis Support Group)
BM Cry-Sis
London WC1N 3XX
Tel: 0171 404 5011

CYSTIC FIBROSIS
The CF Trust
11 London Road
Bromley
Kent BR1 1BY
Tel: 0181 464 7211
Web site: www.cftrust.org.uk

COELIAC DISEASE
The Coeliac Society
PO Box 220
High Wycombe
Bucks HP11 2HY
Tel: 01494 437278
Web Site: www.coeliac.co.uk

DIABETES
The British Diabetic Association
10 Queen Anne Street
London W1M 0BD
Careline: 0171 636 6112

DOWN'S SYNDROME
Down's Syndrome Association
155 Mitcham Road
London SW17 9PG
Tel: 0181 682 4001

Useful Organizations

ECZEMA
National Eczema Society
163 Eversholt Street
London NW1 1BU
Tel: 0171 388 4097
Web site: www.eczema.org

EPILEPSY
British Epilepsy Association
Anstey House
40 Hanover Square
Leeds LS3 1BE
Helpline: 0800 30 90 30

FIRST AID
Contact the following
organizations directly for details
of where and how
you can take part in a first-aid
course near you:

British Red Cross
National Headquarters
9 Grosvenor Crescent
London SW1X 7EJ
Tel: 0171 235 5454

St John Ambulance
1 Grosvenor Crescent
London SW1X 7EE
Tel: 0171 235 5231

St Andrew's Ambulance
Association
48 Milton Street
Glasgow G4 0HR
Tel: 0141 332 4031

GENERAL
Parentline
Endway House
Endway
Hadleigh
Essex SS7 2AN
Helpline: 01702 559900

HEART PROBLEMS
The British Heart Foundation
14 Fitzhardinge Street
London W1H 4DH
Tel: 0171 935 0185

HYPERACTIVITY
The Hyperactive Children's
Support Group
71 Whyke Lane
Chichester
West Sussex PO19 2LD
Tel: 01903 725182

INFANT DEATHS
Foundation for the Study of
Infant Deaths
14 Halkin Street
London SW1X 7DP
24-hour helpline: 0171 235 1721

MENINGITIS
Meningitis Research Foundation
13 High Street
Thornbury
Bristol BS35 2AE
24-hour helpline: 0808 800 3344

Useful Organizations

The National Meningitis Trust
Fern House
Stroud
Gloucs GL5 3TJ
24 hour support line: 0845 6000
800

MIGRAINE
The Migraine Trust
45 Great Ormond Street
London WC1N 3HZ
Tel: 0171 831 4818

STILLBIRTH
SANDS – Stillbirth and Neonatal
Death Society
28 Portland Place
London W1N 4DE
Tel: 0171 436 5881

Index

Index

Index

Index

Index

Index

Acknowledgements

I would like to thank Penelope Cream, Jayne Marsden and Mary Remnant for their tireless energy, encouragement, enthusiasm and attention to detail in guiding the development and production of this book. I would also like to thank my secretary, Cherry Taylor, for her invaluable assistance. Carole Blake, my agent for many years, continues to be a remarkable source of support, and my wife, Barbara, not only provided invaluable advice, but was astonishingly tolerant of the long hours I spent at the word processor.

Last, but definitely not least, I need to thank my children, Katy and Chris, who taught me what practical parenthood is really all about. My thanks to them all.

David Haslam

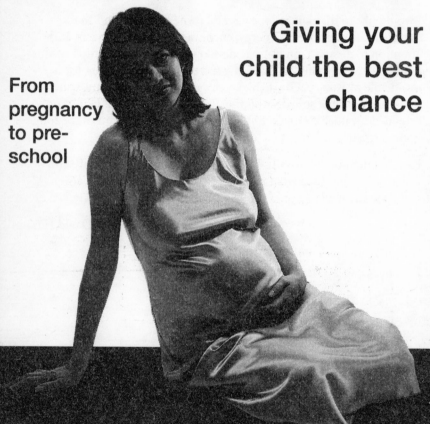